KEY TOPICS IN
OBSTETRICS AND GYNAECOLOGY

Second Edition

The KEY TOPICS Series

Advisors:

T.M. Craft *Department of Anaesthesia and Intensive Care, Royal United Hospital, Bath, UK*
C.S. Garrard *Intensive Therapy Unit, John Radcliffe Hospital, Oxford, UK*
P.M. Upton *Department of Anaesthetics, Treliske Hospital, Truro, UK*

Anaesthesia, Second Edition

Obstetrics and Gynaecology, Second Edition

Accident and Emergency Medicine

Paediatrics

Orthopaedic Surgery

Otolaryngology and Head and Neck Surgery

Ophthalmology

Psychiatry

General Surgery

Renal Medicine

Trauma

Chronic Pain

Oral and Maxillofacial Surgery

Oncology

Forthcoming titles include:

Cardiovascular Medicine

Neonatology

Critical Care

Orthopaedic Trauma Surgery

Respiratory Medicine

Thoracic Surgery

KEY TOPICS IN
OBSTETRICS AND GYNAECOLOGY

Second Edition

R.J. SLADE
FRCS(Glas.), MRCOG
*Consultant Obstetrician and Gynaecologist, Hope Hospital, Salford, UK
and Consultant Gynaecological Surgeon, Christie Hospital,
Manchester, UK*

E. LAIRD
MRCOG, MRNZCOG
*Consultant Obstetrician and Gynaecologist, The Horton General
Hospital, Banbury, UK*

G. BEYNON
FRCS (Ed), MRCOG
*Consultant Obstetrician and Gynaecologist, Princess Anne Hospital,
Southampton and St. Mary's Hospital, Portsmouth, UK*

A. PICKERSGILL
MRCOG
*Lecturer in Obstetrics and Gynaecology, University of Manchester,
Manchester, UK*

βIOS
SCIENTIFIC
PUBLISHERS

Oxford • Washington DC

© BIOS Scientific Publishers Limited, 1998

First published 1993 (ISBN 1 872748 07 4)
Second Edition 1998 (ISBN 1 859962 26 2)

A CIP catalogue record for this book is available from the British Library.

ISBN 1 859962 26 2

BIOS Scientific Publishers Ltd
9 Newtec Place, Magdalen Road, Oxford OX4 1RE, UK
Tel. +44 (0)1865 726286. Fax. +44 (0)1865 246823
World Wide Web home page: http://www.bios.co.uk/

DISTRIBUTORS

Australia and New Zealand
    Blackwell Science Asia
    54 University Street
    Carlton, South Victoria 3053

India
    Viva Books Private Limited
    4325/3 Ansari Road, Daryaganj
    New Delhi 110002

Singapore and South East Asia
    Toppan Company (S) PTE Ltd
    38 Liu Fang Road, Jurong
    Singapore 2262

USA and Canada
    BIOS Scientific Publishers
    PO Box 605, Herndon
    VA 20172-0605

Important Note from the Publisher
The information contained within this book was obtained by BIOS Scientific Publishers Ltd from sources believed by us to be reliable. However, while every effort has been made to ensure its accuracy, no responsibility for loss or injury whatsoever occasioned to any person acting or refraining from action as a result of information contained herein can be accepted by the authors or publishers.

The reader should remember that medicine is a constantly evolving science and while the authors and publishers have ensured that all dosages, applications and practices are based on current indications, there may be specific practices which differ between communities. You should always follow the guidelines laid down by the manufacturers of specific products and the relevant authorities in the country in which you are practising.

Production Editor: Andrea Bosher.
Typeset by Chandos Electronic Publishing, Stanton Harcourt, UK.
Printed by Redwood Books, Trowbridge, UK.

CONTENTS

GYNAECOLOGY

OBSTETRICS

ABBREVIATIONS

A	androstenedione
AC	abdominal circumference
ACTH	adrenocorticotrophic hormone
AFP	alphafeto protein
AFV	amniotic fluid volume
AID	artificial insemination by donor
AIH	artificial insemination by husband
AP	anteroposterior
APCR	activated protein C resistance
APH	antepartum haemorrhage
ARDS	adult respiratory distress syndrome
ARM	artificial rupture of the membranes
BD	two times per day
BP	blood pressure
BPD	biparietal diameter
BPP	biophysical profile
BSO	bilateral salpingo-uophorectomy
cAMP	cyclic adenyl monophosphate
CESDI	confidential enquiry into stillbirths in infancy
CMV	cytomegalovirus
CNS	central nervous system
CPD	cephalopelvic disproportion
CPR	cardiopulmonary resuscitation
CRL	crown rump length
CSF	cerebrospinal fluid
CT	computerized tomography
CTG	cardiotocograph
CVB	chorionic vilus biopsy
CVS	chorionic vilus sampling
CXR	chest X-ray
D&C	dilation and curettage
DHEA	dehyroepiandrosterone
DHEAS	dehyroepiandrosterone sulphate
DIC	disseminated intravascular coagulation
DM	diabetes mellitus
DUB	dysfunctional uterine bleeding
DVT	deep vein thrombosis
ECV	external cephalic version
EFW	estimated fetal weight
ELP	erect lateral pelvimetry

EMG	electromyography
ERPOC	evacuation of retained products of conception
ESR	erythrocyte sedimentation rate
EUA	examination under anaesthetic
FBC	full blood count
FDP	fibrin degradation products
FH	fetal heart
FSH	follicle stimulating hormone
G6PD	glucose-6-phosphate dehydrogenase
GA	general anaesthetic
GFR	glomerular filtration rate
GIFT	gamete intra-fallopian transfer
GIT	gastrointestinal tract
GnRH	gonadotrophin-releasing hormone
GSI	genuine stress incontinence
GSV	gestational sac volume
GTT	glucose tolerance test
HC	head circumference
hCG	human chorionic gonadotrophin
HDL	high density lipoproteins
HLA	human leukocyte
hMG	human menopausal gonadotrophin
HPV	human papilloma virus
HRT	hormone replacement therapy
HSV	herpes simplex virus
HWY	hundred women years
IBS	irritable bowel syndrome
ICSI	intra-cytoplasmic sperm injection
IM	intramuscular
IOL	induction of labour
IPI	intra-peritoneal insemination
ITU	intensive therapy unit
IU	international units
IUCD	intrauterine contraceptive device
IUD	intrauterine death
IUGR	intrauterine growth retardation
IUI	intrauterine contraceptive device
IV	intravenous
IVF	in vitro fertilization
IVH	intraventricular haemorrhage
IVP	intavenous pyelogram
LA	local anaesthetic
LAVH	laparoscopically assisted vaginal hysterectomy

LFT	liver function tests
LH	leuteinizing hormone
LHRH	leuteinizing hormone releasing hormone
LSCS	lower segment caesarian section
LUF	luteinized unruptured follicles
MHC	major histocompatibility complex
MIS	minimally invasive surgery
MoM	multiples of the median
MRI	magnetic resonance imaging
MSSU	midstream specimen of urine
NTD	neural tube defect
OA	osteoarthritis
OCP	oral contraceptive pill
OD	optical density
OHSS	ovarian hyperstimulation syndrome
PCOD	polycystic ovarian disease
PCT	post coital test
PE	pulmonary embolus
PET	pre-eclamptic toxaemia
PG	prostaglandin
PGE	prostaglandin E
PGF	prostaglandin F
PID	pelvic inflammatory disease
PIF	prolactin inhibitory factor
PMS	pre-menstrual syndrome
PO	by mouth
POD	pouch of Douglas
POP	progesterone only pill
PPH	post-partum haemorrhage
PPROM	pre-labour rupture of the membranes
PRF	prolactin-releasing factor
prn	as necessary
PROM	premature rupture of the membranes
PTTK	partial thromboplastin and kaolin time
QDS	four times per day
RAMP	rapid action matrix pregnancy test
RDS	respiratory distress syndrome
RPOC	retained products of conception
RSA	recurrent spontaneous abortion
SC	subcutaneous
SHBG	sex hormone binding globulin
SL	sublingual
SLE	systemic lupus erythamatosus

SR	slow retard
SROM	spontaneous rupture of membranes
SVC	superior vena cava
T	testosterone
TCRE	transcervical resection of the endometrium
TDS	three times per day
TENS	transcutaneous electrical nerve stimulation
TFT	thyroid function tests
TOP	termination of pregnancy
TRH	thyrotrophin-releasing hormone
TURP	transurethral resection of the prostate
TVP	trans vaginal ultrasound scan
U&E	urea and electrolytes
UPSI	unprotected sexual intercourse
USS	ultrasound scan
UTI	urinary tract infection
VDRL	venereal disease reference laboratory
VIN	vulval intraepithelial neoplasia
VLBW	very low birth weight babies
VLDL	very low density lipoproteins
VMA	vanillyl mandelic acid
V-V	vesico-vaginal
WCC	white cell count
WHO	World Health Organization
WR	Wasserman reaction
ZIFT	zygote intra-fallopian transfer

PREFACE TO THE SECOND EDITION

It is hard to imagine how quickly changes occur in obstetrics and gynaecology. Certainly when we wrote the first book we did not realize that in 4 years time when we came to update it, that so many chapters would have to be radically re-written and some new chapters introduced.

We have all progressed to different areas of the country and we would like to welcome a new addition to the team Andrew Pickersgill who has written a new chapter and helped update many of the old ones.

As before, the book is aimed at the part II MRCOG examination and we hope that it will be as well received as the first addition by all those who are sitting or about to sit the exam. It will, we hope, also be helpful to candidates taking the DRCOG and to medical students sitting their finals in obstetrics and gynaecology.

We are indebted to Jonathan Ray for his unstinting encouragement and to our families for their patience whilst we completed the second edition.

Richard J. Slade
Euan Laird
Gareth Beynon
Andrew Pickersgill

PREFACE TO THE FIRST EDITION

Common problems occur regularly in all post-graduate examinations. In obstetrics and gynaecology there is no exception.

This book is aimed at people preparing to take their part II MRCOG. It is prepared as a primer for the exam and should be read as a revision text after more in-depth reading has been performed. Candidates for the DRCOG and medical students sitting their final MB should also find the book useful.

The basis of the book is taken from our revision notes that were compiled when we sat the exam in 1991. Any changes in current practice have been incorporated into the text since we have taken the exam.

The book is divided into Key Topics, so that each area can be read at an individual sitting. Topics were chosen that are regarded as essential knowledge necessary to pass the MRCOG.

The text is designed to be easy to read and very compact as in keeping with the first book in the series *Key Topics in Anaesthesia*. It is expected that the reader should have a basic knowledge of obstetrics and gynaecology before reading this book, as more general aspects of the subject are assumed knowledge.

We would like to thank all our consultants past and present for the encouragement and support they have given us.

We were first introduced to each other at the Christmas 1990 Whipps Cross MRCOG part II course by Roger Baldwin, whose enthusiasm for teaching has been an inspiration to us throughout the writing of this book.

We are indebted to our publishers BIOS, particularly Jonathan Ray and the series editors Tim Craft and Paul Upton for their help and advice.

Finally we would like to thank our respective families for all their continual encouragement, support and patience throughout the writing and preparation of this book.

Richard J. Slade
Euan Laird
Gareth Beynon

ABDOMINAL VERSUS VAGINAL HYSTERECTOMY

Hysterectomy via any route is still the treatment of choice for intractable menorrhagia. One in 5 women under the age of 55 in England and Wales will require a hysterectomy, in USA it is approximately 1 in 3. There is a dichotomy of opinion as to which route is preferable, the incidence of vaginal to abdominal is approximately 1:4 overall.

Abdominal hysterectomy

First performed by Charles Clay in Manchester in 1844. It is still the commonest method in the UK of performing a hysterectomy. It is the operation of choice for the following:

- Fibroids >14 week size.
- Concurrent ovarian pathology where ovarian removal is predicted.
- No descent on examination (nulliparous).
- Laparotomy indicated.
- Malignancy.

In 1985 no fewer than 18 600 hysterectomies were performed for menstrual disorders; the majority were done abdominally. A total of 95% of women questioned after having a hysterectomy were found to be satisfied with the results. Mortality is 4.1–14.6/10 000 with a morbidity of 25–50%.

Vaginal hysterectomy

First described by Langenbeck in 1813. It is a less commonly performed procedure. It is the operation of choice for the following:

(a) Menorrhagia with adequate descent (multiparous).
(b) Prolapse.
(c) Menorrhagia with concurrent prolapse.

Vaginal hysterectomy is the treatment of choice for prolapse, particularly procidentia. Sadly it is performed rarely for menstrual problems. Once a woman has had a single normal delivery it is usually possible to perform a vaginal hysterectomy. Mortality is similar to abdominal hysterectomy, but the morbidity is only 15–20%.

Discussion

This will be limited to treatment for menstrual disorders. An American study showed women who underwent abdominal hysterectomy were older than those undergoing it vaginally.

Ovarian removal at the time of hysterectomy is contentious, unnecessary removal of normal organs versus prophylaxis against malignant change. A total of 95–99% of ovaries can also be removed vaginally if so required. There is still a definite mortality rate from hysterectomy, so other treatments should be considered. The overall complication rate for women undergoing an abdominal hysterectomy was 42.8/100 women, compared with only 24.5/100 women in those who underwent a vaginal hysterectomy. The commonest complication of the vaginal group was urinary retention and/or infection, where as urinary retention, ileus, atelectasis and wound infection and/or dehiscence were found in the abdominal group.

The febrile morbidity rate was twice as common in abdominal hysterectomies as compared to vaginal hysterectomies.

Unintended major surgical procedures such as repair to bowel and bladder trauma were seen more often in vaginal hysterectomies, although rarely.

Ureteric transection only occurred in abdominal hysterectomies as did pulmonary emboli.

The average hospital stay for a vaginal hysterectomy was shortest, with some women able to go home 72 hours after their operation, whereas those who undergo an abdominal procedure stay for at least 7 days.

The major reported complication of vault prolapse occurs in up to 2% of vaginal hysterectomy. Careful apposition of the utero-sacral ligaments during closure minimizes this long-term risk. However, vault prolapse can also occur if an abdominal procedure has been performed.

In the author's (R.J.S.) view, the argument for performing a vaginal hysterectomy instead of an abdominal procedure for menstrual problems is very strong. Not only is it quicker both surgically and in the convalescent period, it is associated with fewer complications, and considerable savings in medical care costs can be made. Whichever way is chosen prophylactic antibiotics should be prescribed.

Further reading

Davies A, O'Connor H, Magos A. A prospective study to evaluate oophorectomy at the time of vaginal hysterectomy. *British Journal of Obstetrics and Gynaecology,* 1996; **103:** 915–20.

Dicker RC *et al.* Complications of abdominal and vaginal hysterectomy among women of reproductive age in the United States. *American Journal of Obstetrics and Gynecology,* 1982; **144:** 841–9.

Shepherd JH. Vaginal hysterectomy. In: Monaghan JM, ed. *Rob and Smith's Operative Surgery.* London: Butterworths, 1987; 79– 92.

Sheth SS. Vaginal hysterectomy. In: Studd J, ed. *Progress in Obstetrics and Gynaecology,* Vol 10. Edinburgh: Churchill Livingstone, 1993; 317–40.

Related topics of interest

Menorrhagia – I (p. 75)
Menorrhagia – II (p. 78)
Minimally invasive surgery (p. 84)

ABNORMALITY OF GENITAL TRACT

Female genital tract congenital abnormality

Congenital abnormalities of the genito-urinary tract are seen in 3–4% of the population and they commonly coexist. Any abnormality in the reproductive tract should be an indication to establish the anatomy of the renal tract.

Vaginal

1. Vaginal agenesis. This occurs in 1:10 000, with 40–50% having associated genito-urinary anomalies. The diagnosis is indicated by primary amenorrhoea and normal secondary sexual characteristics. Testicular feminization needs to be excluded and upper tract USS and/or IVU is indicated. If a uterus is present an abdominal mass (haematometra) and pain will be present at puberty. Formation of a neovagina by repetitive dilatation to the Müllerian pit, fashioning of a perineal pouch, tissue expansion vaginoplasty, full-thickness skin flaps or intestinal grafts have all been described. Such management should be delayed until menstruation demands it.

2. Vaginal atresia. Primary amenorrhoea is the commonest presentation. Haematocolpos should be should be drained in theatre. USS and/or laparoscopy is indicated if there is associated haematosalpinx. Upper vaginal atresia may require an abdominoperineal approach.

3. Vaginal duplication or septae. This occurs as a result of failure of full Müllerian duct fusion. The condition is harmless and such women have normal sexual function.

Cervical

1. Cervical atresia. This is rare in the presence of a functional uterus and vagina. Formation of a uterovaginal fistula is necessary to prevent haematometra, haematosalpinx, adenomyosis and endometriosis. This is achieved via a laparotomy and only one pregnancy has been described. Hysterectomy is the alternative.

Uterine

2. Cervical duplication. This is associated with uterine didelphis. Ensure that two IUCDs are used if this is the chosen method of contraception and that two cervical smears are performed.

1. Uterine agenesis. This presents as primary amenorrhoea and will occur in conjunction with an absent cervix and upper vagina. It is caused by failure of development of the Müllerian ducts. A vestigial uterus and cervix may be present without evidence of a cavity or canal. The vagina in such women is usually shorter than normal, but is adequate for intercourse.

2. Uterine fusion variants. True Müllerian duct duplication on both sides is rare. Variants are common and include uterus didelphis, bicornuate uterus, rudimentary horn (communicating and non-communicating) and subseptate uterus. Most variants are innocuous if menstrual flow can occur. They are associated with an increase in spontaneous abortion, fetal malpresentation, IUGR and abnormalities of placentation.

Fallopian tubes

Hydatid cysts of Morgagni (paramesonephric remnants) are not uncommon. Torsion is rare. Atresia and undeveloped ostia are very rare.

Ovarian

Lack of ovarian function is due to aplasia or dysgenesis and requires HRT. Dysgenetic ovaries will require excision as up to 30% have malignant potential. Donor ZIFT means that such women can bear children, so hysterectomy is not always an option at oophorectomy in such cases.

Renal

Bilateral renal agenesis is known as Potter's syndrome and is incompatible with life. Unilateral renal agenesis is relatively common. USS will allow a diagnosis. Simple remnants of the pronephros and mesonephros, the epoophoron, paroophoron and Gartner's duct cysts are benign. Other renal anomalies include multiple renal vessels, duplications of the upper tract, ectopic ureters, horseshoe kidneys, congenital bilateral polycystic kidneys (fatal), urachal malformations including fistulae, ectopia vesicae, cloacal exstrophy and rectourinary fistulae.

Ambiguous genitalia

A person with ambiguous external genitalia is known as a hermaphrodite. True hermaphrodites have both ovarian and testicular tissue and are very rare. In pseudo-hermaphroditism, e.g. adrenogenital syndrome due to congenital virilizing adrenal hyperplasia (the commonest form of female hermaphroditism), there is ambiguous genitalia, but the patient's chromatin and karyotype correspond to the gonadal sex.

Intersexual conditions, e.g. testicular feminization, are classified according to the true histology of the gonads. Testicular feminization patients appear to be normal females, but have testes and are genotypically XY. It occurs in 1:50 000 females and is a sex-linked recessive disorder. It presents with primary amenorrhoea and infertility. Patients with mixed gonadal dysgenesis, which is very rare, have a testis on one side, an undifferentiated gonad on the other and sex chromatin-negative nuclei. They may be normal female, intermediate sex or normal male.

All of these conditions require expert examination, biochemical and hormone enzyme assays, karyotyping and referral to the appropriate specialty.

Further reading

Duncan SLB. Embryology of the female genital tract: its genetic defects and congenital anomalies. In: Shaw RW, Soutter WP, Stanton SL, eds. *Gynaecology.* Edinburgh: Churchill Livingstone, 1992: 3–21.

Moore KL. *The Developing Human*, 2nd edn. Philadelphia: WB Saunders, 1977.

Related topics of interest

ABORTION SPONTANEOUS/RECURRENT

In the UK a spontaneous abortion is defined as a pregnancy loss occurring before 24 completed weeks of gestation. The WHO definition is 'the loss of a fetus or embryo weighing 500 g or less which corresponds to a gestational age of 20–22 weeks, the irreducible age for fetal well-being'. 16–25% of all women will experience vaginal bleeding in early pregnancy. It is followed by a live birth in 50% of affected pregnancies. 25% of all women will experience at least one miscarriage. The actual incidence of spontaneous abortion is unknown, but figures greater than 30% of all conceptions are reported. A woman who has three consecutive abortions is deemed to be a recurrent aborter.

Causes

1. *Chromosomal anomalies.* Up to 50% of first trimester abortions are chromosomally abnormal.

2. *Placental abnormalities.* Utero-placental ischaemia and retroplacental haemorrhage have been reported.

3. *Infection.* Commonest are *Listeria monocytogenes, Campylobacter* spp, *Brucella* spp, CMV, *Rubella* and *Herpes simplex.*

4. *Uterine.* Congenital anomalies.

5. *Endocrine.* Luteal insufficiency, PCOS.

6. *Immunological.* Autoimune (SLE).

7. *Undetermined.* 25% of cases no cause is found.

Spontaneous abortion presents in a number of ways:

- Threatened abortion: bleeding, minimal pain, closed cervix and a viable pregnancy.
- Missed abortion: failure of embryonic growth in spite of placental viability. Associated with a brown discharge, disappearance of pregnancy symptoms, a uterus smaller than expected and an empty sac on USS.
- Inevitable abortion: bleeding with clots, pain, an open cervix and a non-viable pregnancy.
- Incomplete abortion:bleeding with RPOC seen on USS.

- Complete abortion: no bleeding, closed cervix, empty uterus on USS and therefore no treatment. (*Ectopic pregnancy must have been excluded*).
- Septic abortion: Infected incomplete abortion, pain, bleeding, pyrexia *E. coli, Bacteroides* spp, *Cl. welchi* and streptococci. IV antibiotics must be given prior to evacuation.

Management

The management of threatened abortion is rest followed by USS to confirm viability. No treatment has been shown to be effective. The risk of abortion following a positive ultrasound showing a fetal heart is less than 5%.

Septic abortion must be treated by surgical evacuation and antibiotics. Complications are very rare, although the mortality rate is 12.5 per million usually resulting from haemorrhage or infection. The major morbidity is the rare occurrence of Asherman's syndrome following evacuation and also the potential psychological effects of the abortion on the woman.

Surgical evacuation is no longer the only method of emptying a uterus in other types of abortion (incomplete or missed). Medical management using *mifepristone* (antiprogestogen) and *misoprostol* (PGE_1 analogue) in a regimen of 600 µg orally followed 36–48 hours later by 400 µg of misoprostol and 200 µg 2 hours later has been shown to achieve complete uterine evacuation in 95% of cases of miscarriage under 12 weeks.

Expectant management is effective for incomplete abortions, but the woman may bleed for up to 1 week.

Recurrent spontaneous abortion

The incidence of three consecutive abortions is approximately 1%. Assuming 12–15% of pregnancies miscarry the expected chance of three consecutive pregnancy losses would be lower at 0.3%. A simple scheme for investigations is shown:

1. History/examination.

2. Genetic. Parental/fetal karyotype. Parental chromosome abnormality is found in 3–5%; the most common abnormality is a Robertsonian translocation.

3. *Anatomical.* Laparoscopy/hysteroscopy/cervical incompetence (10–15% chance).

4. *Infective.* Antibody titre, endometrial biopsy, TB. Bacterial vaginosis is found in 22% late miscarriages.

5. *Systemic.* GTT, poorly controlled diabetes with raised HbA1C is associated with an increased risk of abortion.

6. *Endocrine.* LH levels in first half cycle (PCOS). 11% hypersecrete LH. Also there is a 1–2% premature menopause rate.

7. *Immunological.* Anti-phospholipidantibodies (aPl) – 15% of women with recurrent miscarriage will have persistently positive test for aPl, with only a 10% birth rate without treatment. Lupus anticoagulant, cardiolipin, autoantibody screening, compliment levels, HLA typing.

8. *Thrombophilic.* Activated protein C resistance (APCR).

It must be remembered that 70% of patients will have a spontaneous resolution and 75–81% will attain a pregnancy with just psychological supportive treatment. There is no evidence that exogenous progestogens or hCG are effective in preventing miscarriage.

Various methods of treatment have been tried such as low dose aspirin, prednisolone, subcutaneous heparin and immunotherapy. Low dose aspirin (75 mg daily) and unfractioned heparin (5000 IU BD) have been used successfully in women with aPl. The use of both is more effective than aspirin alone (71% vs. 42% live birth rate) although by using heparin there is an associated decrease in maternal spinal bone density (5.4%).

The discovery of a raised LH in the follicular phase results in premature completion of oocyte maturation resulting in poor implantation.

Commonly a raised LH is found in PCOS and also the incidence of PCOS in recurrent aborters was 58% compared to only 22% in normal pregnancies.

It may therefore be possible to predict pregnancy outcome; if the D8 LH>10 IU/l there is a five-fold increase in the likelihood of miscarriage. However, suppression of LH with GnRH analogues does not improve the outcome of women who hypersecrete LH.

Immunological therapy such as blood transfusions containing leukocytes has been shown to increase allograft survival. This led to transfusions in women with idiopathic abortions in a hope of modifying the immune response within the uterus. Early work was encouraging with a success rate of 77%, but the success rate of just psychotherapy alone must be born in mind.

Further reading

Beard RW, Sharp F, eds. *Early Pregnancy Loss: Mechanisms and Treatment*. London: Royal College of Obstetricians and Gynaecologists, 1988.

Chipchase J, James D. Randomised trial of expectant versus surgical management of spontaneous miscarriage. *British Journal of Obstetrics and Gynaecology*, 1997; **104:** 840–1.

Edmonds DK. Spontaneous and recurrent abortion. In: Shaw RW *et al.*, eds. *Gynaecology*, 1992; **15:** 205–18.

Nielson S, Hahlin M. Expectant management of first trimester miscarriage. *Lancet*, 1995; **345:** 84–6.

Rai R, Clifford K, Regan L. The modern preventative treatment of recurrent miscarriage. *British Journal of Obstetrics and Gynaecology*, 1996; **103:** 106–10.

Related topics of interest

Endometriosis (p. 31)
Polycystic ovarian disease (PCOD) (p. 104)
Therapeutic abortion and the Human Fertilization and Embryology Act 1990 (p. 132)

AMENORRHOEA, PRIMARY AND SECONDARY

Primary amenorrhoea

This is defined as absence of menstruation, there being significant delay in the menarche, patients commonly presenting at around age 16 years.

The commonest reason for primary amenorrhoea is delayed puberty; the natural anxiety of the patient and her parents may warrant basic investigations but reassurance may be all that is required.

Normal menstruation depends on normal female pelvic anatomy, with appropriate stimulation of the pelvic target organs by the relevant hormones, in association with an appropriate ponderal index.

Two X chromosomes are necessary for ovarian development and maintenance of the menstrual cycle.

Diagnosis

1. *History.* Cyclical pain may suggest anatomical obstruction to menstrual flow, or there may be an element of virilization, either at birth or at puberty, or a history of chronic severe illness or weight loss and heavy exercise.

2. *Examination.* A general examination is performed noting the development of secondary sexual characteristics and the height of the patient, and looking for specific features, e.g. those suggestive of Turner's syndrome.

An examination under anaesthesia may reveal an anatomical cause.

3. *Investigation.* This should begin with karyotyping and all chromosomal anomalies should be further investigated.

Pituitary hormones may be reduced as a result of primary or secondary pituitary failure, e.g. craniopharyngioma, or inhibited by raised adrenal steroid production. Ovarian failure or maldevelopment causes elevation of pituitary gonadotrophins.

Laparoscopy may be necessary to visualize the pelvic organs and biopsy the ovaries.

Treatment   The aim is to restore normal sexual function and fertility where possible.

Ovarian failure is treated with exogenous sex hormones, pituitary failure with gonadotrophins.

Simple surgery will correct an imperforate hymen.

Successful treatment of absence of the lower genital tract has been achieved with the use of graduated glass dilators with full coital function as a result. Where these measures fail then complex plastic surgery procedures may be necessary in an attempt to achieve satisfactory coitus.

These patients require a great deal of psychological support and adequate counselling facilities must be available.

Phenotypic females, but with non-functioning gonads, be they ovaries or testes, should have these gonads excised because of the high risk of malignant change.

It is unwise to inform the patient and attempt to change the sex of rearing when they are found to be genotypic males.

Secondary amenorrhoea

This is defined as an absence of menstruation for 6 months or more in a previously normal female of reproductive years that is not the result of pregnancy, lactation or hysterectomy. Causes include long-term treatment with hormones such as Depo-Provera, danazol or gonadotrophin-releasing hormone analogues.

Any severe illness may result in amenorrhoea and this should be excluded before definitive investigation is undertaken.

Diagnosis   *1. History.* There may be a family history of premature menopause. Presentation may be preceded by a period of oral contraceptive usage or severe weight loss, associated with diet, anorexia nervosa or depression. Heavy exercise is associated with amenorrhoea and stress may be a factor.

A hormonal cause may be suggested by galactorrhoea or virilizing symptoms.

An obstructive cause is suggested by cyclical pelvic pain and a history of gynaecological or obstetric surgery.

2. Examination. Signs of virilization, nipple discharge, signs of a pituitary tumour (visual field disturbance and papilloedema), a pelvic mass (uterine or ovarian) or an abdominal mass (uterine, ovarian or adrenal) may lead to the diagnosis.

3. Investigation. This is decided by preceding history and examination. The commonest causes are PCOS and premature menopause, which is confirmed by gonadotrophin estimation. A full hormone profile will determine a pituitary or adrenal aetiology and may suggest polycystic ovaries.

Ultrasound or examination under anaesthesia may reveal an ovarian or adrenal cause as well as identifying any site of obstruction to menstrual flow.

Treatment

Treatment is directed to the cause: hormone replacement for premature menopause, gonadotrophin stimulation for hormone-induced amenorrhoea or hypopituitarism (if fertility is desired, otherwise O/C or HRT if oestrogen deficient), counselling and psychiatric treatment for stress-related causes and depression, surgical correction of outflow obstruction and definitive treatment by the relevant specialists for pituitary and adrenal tumours.

Further reading

Edmonds DK. Primary amenorrhoea. In: Studd J, ed. *Progress in Obstetrics and Gynaecology,* Vol. 10. Edinburgh: Churchill Livingstone, 1993: 281–95.

Shearman RS. Primary amenorrhoea. Secondary amenorrhoea. In: Whitfield CR, ed. *Dewhurst's Textbook of Obstetrics and Gynaecology for Postgraduates*, 4th edn. Oxford: Blackwell Scientific Publications, 1986: 63–79.

Related topics of interest

BARTHOLIN'S GLANDS

The pea-sized, mucus-secreting vestibular glands of Bartholin are situated at the opening of the vagina, lying deep to the posterior parts of the labia majora and are usually impalpable. Each drains into the groove between the hymen and the posterior part of the labium minora via a duct which is 3 cm long. Anterior to each gland is the bulb of the vestibule that traverses anteriorly to reach the root of the clitoris.

Problems

- *Infection.*
- *Treatment.*
- *Differential diagnosis.*

1. Infection. Bartholin's gland can respond very well to antibiotics, usually flucloxacillin, but there is a tendency for the infection to recur. Healing in these chronic cases is often by fibrosis with closure of the duct orifice causing cyst formation which can then become infected.

The most common bacteria are staphylococci species, *E. coli* or gonococci, and a swab of the contents is therefore essential.

These type of infections are most common in diabetics, during pregnancy and in immunocompromised patients.

2. Treatment. In the acute abscess case the operation of choice is *marsupialization;* that is, an ellipse of skin over the cyst is removed followed by drainage of the pus. The cyst wall is then apposed to the vaginal skin maintaining an aperture the size of a finger tip to allow for continual drainage and healing from the base upwards.

Excision of the cyst, and more importantly its duct, should only be undertaken between acute episodes in recurrent cases.

3. Differential diagnosis.
(a) *Gartner's duct cysts*: These are remnants of mesonephric origin and are classically found in the paravaginal area usually laterally or antero-laterally. They are usually symptomless and of low tension and can often be missed on vaginal examination.

(b) *Skene's duct cysts*: Otherwise known as periurethral or paraurethral glands, they lie on the floor of the urethra at its lower end. Infection causes dysuria, and compression may cause pus to exude into the urethra.

(c) *Retention cysts*: These are of a variety of origins and may occur such sebaceous, epidermoid, implantation dermoid and clitoral cysts.

(d) *Others*: For example, such as fibroma, lipoma, haemangioma, neurofibroma and hidradenoma.

(e) *Carcinoma of Bartholin's gland*: This rare carcinoma can result in a unilateral swelling and histologically is an adenocarcinoma in most cases. The prognosis is less favourable than squamous carcinoma of the vulva, due to its developing deep in the vulva, and diagnosis may be delayed.

Further reading

Evans AS. Marsupialization or excision of a Bartholin cyst. In: *Rob and Smith's Operative Surgery*. Monaghan JM, ed. 1987: 25–8.

Related topics of interest

CANCER OF THE CERVIX

Cervical cancer is a disease which, in a high proportion of cases, goes through a preinvasive phase that is detectable by clinical methods. Efficient screening programmes have been shown to decrease the incidence of invasive cancer.

The advent of computerized call and recall in the national screening programme in 1987 has led to a reduction in the death rate to approximately 1500 cases per year in England and Wales.

The reduction in incidence is less marked as there is an increased tendency to recognize microinvasive disease (Stage Ia).

Aetiology

Transmission of human papillomavirus subtypes 16, 18, 31, 33 and 35 by sexual intercourse is the prime factor in the aetiology of cervical cancer. Associated factors include smoking, increased parity, low social class, use of the oral contraceptive pill and infective agents, especially herpes simplex virus and chlamydia.

Age

The peak incidence of development of invasive cancer of the cervix occurs in the fifth and sixth decades of life. The actual incidence in this age group has been declining in most countries with an effective screening programme. At the same time, however, there has been a marked increase in the incidence in younger women, particularly in the 25–35 age group. In this group there is a higher proportion of adenocarcinoma (up to 26%, compared with an overall incidence of 10%).

Pathology

Squamous carcinoma accounts for around 90% of cancers of the cervix. A high proportion appear to contain DNA from the HPV-16 and -18 viruses incorporated in the host cell nuclear DNA. The degree of differentiation and presence of keratinization influences the prognosis, with small-cell, non-keratinizing tumours having a poor outlook.

Adenocarcinoma accounts for the majority of the remainder. Mixed adeno and squamous tumours may coexist.

Clinical features

Early invasive cancers may be detected by colposcopy and biopsy. Presenting symptoms are irregular or post-menopausal bleeding and vaginal discharge which may be offensive.

Vaginal examination reveals a mass or ulcer on the cervix, and the diagnosis is confirmed by biopsy of the lesion and the disease staged at examination under anaesthesia with cystoscopy, and, where appropriate, sigmoidoscopy.

Spread of the disease is by direct infiltration of adjacent structures and via lymphatics to the regional pelvic and then para-aortic nodes. The supraclavicular group may be involved as a late manifestation of disease. Bloodstream spread is a rare, late phenomenon, usually involving lungs and liver.

Treatment is governed by the staging of the disease: radical hysterectomy with bilateral pelvic lymphadenectomy is the operation of choice for stage 1 and early stage 2 disease. Radiotherapy gives similar results but the side-effect profile is such that surgery is the preferred option in the majority of cases. Radiotherapy is the primary treatment in late-stage disease and is given after surgery when there is lymph node spread or a large or incompletely excised primary. Combination chemotherapy may cause significant tumour shrinkage; its usefulness as primary adjuvant therapy awaits further evaluation.

Recurrent disease, if local, is treated with radiotherapy if the patient has not been previously irradiated. If there is a central, mobile recurrence and there is no evidence of distant spread then pelvic exenteration may be performed, with a 50% 5-year survival rate in carefully selected patients. Those not amenable to radical surgery may be treated with chemotherapy: Combination chemotherapy including CIS platinum has shown a clinical response rate of 90%, but very few patients have a long-term response, of the order of 10% at 2 years.

Prognosis

Overall survival in stage 1 disease is over 80%; survival rates of 90% in node-negative patients will drop to 50–60% if pelvic nodes are involved. Other adverse factors include a large primary tumour, lymphatic and vascular space involvement and poorly differentiated tumours. Five-year survival in stage 2 disease is of the order of 50–60%, stage 3 disease 25–40% and stage 4 around 5–15%.

Early recurrence is associated with a high mortality; 62% of recurrences occur in the first 2 years and 75% within 3 years after treatment of early stage disease.

Further reading

Beral V. Epidemiology and aetiology of cancers of the female genital tract. In: Shepherd JH, Monaghan JM, eds. *Clinical Gynaecological Oncology*, 2nd edn. Oxford: Blackwell Scientific Publications, 1990: 1–16.

Monaghan JM. The management of advanced and recurrent cervical cancer by pelvic exenteration. In: Shepherd JH, Monaghan JM, eds. *Clinical Gynaecological Oncology*, 2nd edn. Oxford: Blackwell Scientific Publications, 1990: 98–114.

Shepherd JH. Cervical cancer: the management of early stage disease. In: Shepherd JH, Monaghan JM, eds. *Clinical Gynaecological Oncology*, 2nd edn. Oxford: Blackwell Scientific Publications, 1990: 64–97.

Related topics of interest

Cancer in pregnancy (p. 182)
Fistulae in obstetrics and gynaecology (p. 38)
Intermenstrual, post-coital and post-menopausal bleeding (p. 65)
Perioperative complications in obstetrics and gynaecology (p. 100)
Premalignant disease of the cervix (p. 108)
Radiotherapy (p. 119)

CHRONIC PELVIC PAIN

Over one third of outpatient referrals to a gynaecologist is for pelvic pain, the majority do not have gross pelvic pathology.

The differential diagnosis is between *gynaecological* and *non-gynaecological* causes:

Gynaecological
- Chronic pelvic inflammatory disease.
- Cyclical pain – dysmenorrhoea, *mittelschmertz*.
- Endometriosis.
- Neoplasia – benign conditions, e.g. ovarian cysts, fibroids.
- Pelvic pain syndrome (venous congestion).
- PCOD.
- Utero-vaginal prolapse.
- Residual ovary syndrome – symptoms from ovaries left at the time of hysterectomy; 75% will present with pain.

Non-gynaecological
- GIT – diverticulitis, inflammatory bowel disease, IBS, obstruction.
- Urinary tract – calculus, infection, retention, malignancy.
- Musculo-skeletal – lumbo-sacral OA, prolapsed disc.

Investigations

Laparoscopy is the usual investigation. Over 50% of laparoscopies each year are performed for pelvic pain. Prior to laparascopy, a USS is often useful in that it is a non-invasive method of detecting pelvic masses and also PCOS. Using the Doppler mode on a scan, it is also possible to measure the diameter of the pelvic veins.

X-rays are often indicated such as a plain X-ray of the lumbo-sacral spine and hips; IVP, barium enema and transuterine pelvic venography may be necessary.

Treatment

Each specific gynaecological pathology must be treated along standard lines. However in many women with chronic pelvic pain, no clearly defined pathological cause will be found. This may be associated with pelvic venous congestion or a non-gynaecological cause. In the absence of a diagnosis, reassurance is extremely important. Patient symptoms are very helpful.

Symptoms suggestive of irritable bowel syndrome include: diarrhoea/constipation; episodes of pain more than once a month; relief of pain with defecation and abdominal distension.

Symptoms suggestive of pelvic congestion are: deep dyspareunia and post-coital aching; pain of variable nature and location; exacerbation on standing; relieved on lying and radiating through to back or down legs.

Pelvic venous congestion is restricted to women in their reproductive years and is characterized by a dull aching pain with acute exacerbations. It is commonly in the lower abdomen, but can go into either iliac fossa. It is also associated with dysmenorrhoea, deep dyspareunia and post-coital discomfort.

The treatment of pelvic venous congestion can be by hysterectomy which results in almost universal cure. Pharmacological treatment is with continuous high dose progestogens (medroxy progesterone acetate 30–50 mg/day) which will suppress ovulation. This has achieved good short term success, but no long term benefit. The use of ergot alkaloids to relieve the pain by selective venoconstriction has proven to be successful for 48 hours post injection, but has no long term benefit.

Psychotherapy is effective in this group of women along with careful explanation of the problem.

A negative laparoscopy may provide reassurance and symptoms may resolve.

Further reading

Farthing MJG. Irritable bowel, irritable body or irritable brain? *British Medical Journal,* 1995, **310:** 171–5.

Frappell J, Stanton SL. Chronic pelvic pain. In: Studd J, ed. *Progress in Obstetrics and Gynaecology,* Vol. 9. Edinburgh: Churchill Livingstone. 1991; **15:** 245–58.

Manning AP, Thompson WG, Heaton KW, Morris AF. Towards positive diagnosis of the irritable bowel. *British Medical Journal,* 1978, 653–4.

Reginald PW, Pearce S, Beard RW. Pelvic pain due to venous congestion. In: Studd J, ed. *Progress in Obstetrics and Gynaecology,* Vol. 7. Edinburgh: Churchill Livingstone. 1989; **18:** 275–92.

Related topics of interest

Abdominal pain in pregnancy (p. 154)
Dyspareunia (p. 26)
Endometriosis (p. 31)
Infection in pregnancy (p. 232)
Pelvic inflammatory disease (p. 96)

CONTRACEPTION AND STERILIZATION

The ideal contraceptive (100% effective, completely reversible, totally acceptable and absolutely free of side-effects) does not exist. Contraceptive effectiveness is expressed in the number of pregnancies per hundred women-years (HWY) and is known as the Pearl Index.

Relative methods of contraception

Rhythm
The time of maximum fertility (i.e. the 3–4 days around ovulation) is predicted from previous menstrual calendars, temperature charting or ovulation prediction kits, and abstenance of intercourse. The effectiveness is of the order of 25 HWY.

Coitus interruptus
This is still widely practised and has a failure rate of at least 20 HWY.

Barrier methods
These work on the principle of preventing the sperm gaining access to the upper genital tract. They also have a role to play in decreasing the spread of sexually transmitted disease. Used with a spermicide they have an effectiveness of 7–20 HWY. They include female and male condoms, diaphragms and cervical caps, and must be used before penetration occurs.

Intrauterine contraceptive devices (IUCDs)
Their major action is to interfere with blastocyst implantation. They may be inert, copper-based, or medicated. They are associated with menstrual irregularity, pain, uterine perforation, pelvic infection, ectopic pregnancy, spontaneous abortion and preterm delivery. They can be used as a post-coital contraceptive if inserted within 72 hours of unprotected sexual intercourse (UPSI). They have an effectiveness of 2–5 HWY and are best fitted after menstruation. They can be left *in situ* for 3–5 years, and in a woman of >40 years may be left until the menopause. The latest device on the market known as the MIRENA System, has secondary amenorrhoea (85% at 6 months) as a useful side-effect.

Oral contraceptive pill (OCP)
1. Combined OCP. The dominant mode of action of combined OCPs (oestrogen and progestogen) is

inhibition of the midcycle LH peak and thus inhibition of ovulation. The oestrogen content ranges from 20 to 50 μg. The progestogens can be classified into two groups: those containing or metabolized to norethisterone and those containing norgestrel or its close relative desogestrel. Phased formulations more closely mimic endogenous cyclical hormonal activity. OCPs carry a risk of thromboembolism and cardiovascular complications, and these risks escalate with age, obesity, cigarette smoking, diabetes, hypertension and familial hyperlipidaemia. Effectiveness is limited by vomiting and diarrhoea, some antibiotics and hepatic enzyme-inducing drugs. They may cause weight gain, mood disturbance, loss of libido and lactation failure; it is recommended that they are started 3–4 weeks post-partum for contraception. If breakthrough bleeding occurs, a higher dose may be indicated. Discontinue them for 4 weeks before major elective surgery and leg surgery. When not discontinued before major surgery, subcutaneous heparin prophylaxis should be employed. Their use is associated with a reduction in the incidence of endometrial and ovarian malignancy, and with an increase in cervical intraepithelial neoplasia, cervical malignancy and hepatic malignancy. They may be associated with an increase in breast malignancy if used for more than 5 years before the first pregnancy, and may also cause acute intermittent porphyria. Absolute contraindications to their use include breast cancer, DVT and PE, active liver disease, rifampicin treatment, familial hyperlipidaemia and pregnancy. They have an effectiveness of <1 HWY if used corrrectly. They can be used as emergency post-coital protection, i.e. morning after pill (MAP) <72 hours from UPSI, in a regimen of two 50 μg tablets immediately and two tablets 12 hours later. Future fertility can be diminished. Up to 12 months of post-pill amenorrhoea is seen in 6/1000 users.

2. *Progestogen-only pill (POP).* The POP does not always inhibit ovulation. It enhances cervical mucus hostility towards sperm. It is suitable for older patients with contraindications to oestrogen use, and the

younger motivated patient. They have a higher failure rate than combined OCPs, and need to be taken at the same time each day. Efficacy is decreased if the time of taking is delayed by >3 hours. Menstrual irregularities are more common. They do not inhibit lactation.

Depot injection

Medroxy progesterone acetate, 150 mg (Depo-Provera), is a long-acting (3 months) progestogen given by IM injection. It is almost as effective as combined OCPs. It can cause complete amenorrhoea, transient infertility, bleeding and cycle irregularity after discontinuation. It is useful as a short-term measure. It does not inhibit lactation, but may cause increased bleeding if given very early in the puerperium.

MAP

This has already been described above. Trials are being carried out to evaluate mifepristone (RU 486) as a MAP.

Absolute methods of contraception

All women and men seeking sterilization should undergo counselling. The failure rate, irreversibility, advantages of laparoscopy vs. laparotomy, menstrual outcome and vasectomy should be included in the counselling.

Female sterilization

This is performed surgically in a variety of ways, either laparoscopically or by laparotomy. General anaesthesia is usually required. There is a failure rate of the order of 1:500–2000. The highest failure rates are amongst those performed at Caesarean section or those done in the immediate puerperium. There are no endocrine changes after sterilization, but the procedure is associated rarely with the development of peritubal adhesions, pelvic pain and infection. Reversal of female sterilization is associated with a successful pregnancy rate of >50%.

Male sterilization

Vasectomy is a safer surgical procedure, in that it can be easily and painlessly performed under local anaesthesia and does not carry the risks associated with entering the peritoneal cavity as is necessary for female sterilization. After vasectomy it is essential to get a laboratory-negative sperm count, on two occasions, before assuming sterility. Antisperm antibodies may develop after vasectomy, and have been linked with continued sterility after vasectomy reversal (which is surgically successful in 50–70% of cases). There are no other demonstrable endocrine, libido or potency changes after vasectomy. The failure rate is 1–4:1000 owing to vas recanalization.

Further reading

Newton J. Contraception, sterilization and abortion. In: Shaw RW, Soutter, WP, Stanton SL. *Gynaecology*. Edinburgh: Churchill Livingstone, 1992: 291–312.

Related topics of interest

Hormone replacement therapy (p. 50)
Therapeutic Abortion and The Human Fertilisation and Embryology Act 1990 (p. 132)

DYSPAREUNIA

Dyspareunia is defined as painful sexual intercourse. It can be divided into two distinct groups. *Superficial* is defined as introital pain and *deep* is defined as pelvic pain.

It must be differentiated from vaginismus which is due to spasm of the pubo-coccygeus muscle leading to closure of the vaginal introitus, preventing penetration.

Superficial

1. Vulval causes

- Infective – HSV/HPV.
- Vulval dystrophy.
- Traumatic.
- Atrophic.
- Vulval carcinoma.

2. Vaginal causes

- Congenital – stenosis/bands.
- Infective – HSV/HPV/candida.
- Bechet's syndrome.
- Bartholin's cysts/abscess.
- Urethral caruncle.
- Fistula.
- Vaginal carcinoma.

Deep

1. Cervical

- Infective – specifically HSV.
- Carcinoma.

2. Uterus

- Endometritis: *E. coli*, chlamydia, anaerobic streptococci etc.
- Adenomyosis.
- Retroversion – secondary to any cause (endometriosis, fibroids, PID).

3. Adnexae

- Ovaries prolapsed into the POD due to retroversion.
- Endometriosis.
- Ovarian cysts.

- PID.
- Ectopic gestation.
- Hydrosalpinx.

4. Extra-pelvic

- Appendicitis.
- Inflammatory bowel disease.
- Diverticular disease.
- TB.
- Constipation.
- Irritable bowel syndrome.

Laparoscopy is the investigation of choice for deep dyspareunia.

If all these logical causes have been ruled out (and appropriately treated) then the more difficult diagnosis of dyspareunia secondary to a psychosexual cause may be made and expert counselling should be introduced.

Further reading

Kolodny RC, Masters WH, Johnson VE. *Textbook of Sexual Medicine.* Boston: Little, Brown, 1979.

Related topics of interest

Endometriosis (p. 31)
Pelvic inflammatory disease (p. 96)

ECTOPIC PREGNANCY

Ectopic pregnancy is defined as the implantation of a pregnancy outside the uterine cavity. The incidence ranges from 1:28 births in Jamaica (a hospital only population) to 1:130 in the USA. There were 8 deaths from ectopic pregnancy during the triennia 1991–1993, the death rate being 0.3/1000.

The commonest site is the ampulla of the Fallopian tube followed by other sites within the tube, the isthmus, the fimbrial end and the cornua; these constitute 98% of the total. Other sites include the ovary, cervix, broad ligament and the abdomen.

Predisposing factors

- Pelvic inflammatory disease – chlamydia, gonorrhoea.
- Previous ectopic pregnancy.
- Congenital anomalies, e.g. diverticulae.
- Progestogen only contraceptives. If pregnancy occurs it is more likely to be ectopic, although the ectopic rates are no higher than those using no contraceptive.
- Levenorgatrel-releasing intrauterine system.
- Previous tubal surgery, e.g. sterilization, reanastomosis.
- GIFT and IVF.
- Exposure to diethylstilboestrol *in utero*.
- Non-caucasion and >35 years old.

Diagnosis

Ninety per cent of cases present with pain, 80% have amenorrhoea, 50% experience abnormal vaginal bleeding.

Classically the pain precedes the bleeding (unproved), 25% have symptoms of pregnancy.

Shoulder tip pain occurs in less than 20%, and is associated with rupture.

Signs range from shock and collapse to nothing, cervical excitation with or without lower abdominal pain.

If the history is suggestive of an ectopic pregnancy, an internal examination is contraindicated without course to theatre. With a positive pregnancy test a vaginal USS trans vaginal ultrasound scan (TVS) showing an empty uterus with free fluid with or without adnexal mass. Combining these findings gives a 93% prediction of an ectopic pregnancy. TVS alone may be normal in 25% of cases.

Quantitative βhCG has revolutionized the early diagnosis and helps distinguish ectopic pregnancies from early intrauterine ones and complete abortions.

Radioimmunoassays (detecting βhCG of 5 IU/l) will detect βhCG in serum and urine, 9 and 13 days after ovulation respectively. βhCG will double every 2 days, thus there is a delay of 2 weeks between the biochemical detection of implantation (hCG >10 IU/l) and the visualization of a gestation sac by TVS.

hCG is diagnostic of pregnancy >25 IU/l. At levels of 1000 IU/l a sac should be seen with TVS. Ectopic (and 15% of normal) pregnancies are associated with an increase in titres of hCG of <66% in 2 days. If this happens a laparoscopy should be performed if the TVS is unhelpful.

Culdocentesis/culdoscopy/colpotomy are rarely used in the UK.

Treatment

In shocked patients, immediate resuscitation followed by laparotomy is mandatory. This usually results in salpingectomy to stop haemorrhage.

In a suspected ectopic, a laparoscopy is essential. Laparoscopic surgery is now advocated. It is as safe and effective as a laparotomy, with shorter hospital stay, lower costs and quicker return to work.

Linear salpingostomy and removal of the pregnancy is the operation of choice. Trophoblastic tissue may persist (3–20%), higher than with open surgery. Weekly serum hCG estimations should fall, becoming undetectable within an average of 4 weeks.

Cervical ectopic pregnancy is often not recognized until the pregnancy has been removed by vaginal evacuation, with the patient having presented as an incomplete abortion.

The first sign of a problem is continual heavy bleeding; examination will reveal a sac-like cavity in the cervix with the body of the uterus palpable above.

The most effective treatment is inserting a 14-gauge Foley catheter and inflate the balloon until the locally applied pressure controls the bleeding. Up to 50 ml sterile water can be inserted into the balloon without it bursting. The pressure can be released after 24 hours and the catheter removed.

The catheter will allow blood from above the balloon only to drain. The use of a circumcervical suture is sometimes necessary to prevent the balloon from slipping out.

Hysterectomy has been performed in the past for a cervical ectopic pregnancy.

Sequelae

Over 50% of women who have had an ectopic pregnancy will want to conceive again; only one-third will achieve a live infant.

15% will have another ectopic pregnancy.

The risk of ectopic pregnancy after conservative surgery is 7% after laparoscopy and 14% after laparotomy.

Conservative management of ectopic pregnancy with 50 mg/m^2 IM methotrexate is successful in 92%. Potassium chloride, adrenaline, PGE$_2$ and PGF$_{2\alpha}$ have been successfully injected into gestation sacs.

Methotrexate is advised if the pregnancy is <3.5 cm, unruptured, hCG <1500 IU/l and no evidence of fetal heart (FH) on TVS. βhCG may initially rise (1–4 days) following this procedure but will then fall.

Although a few successes have been reported with the antiprogesteron, mifepristone, results are not consistent and at present it cannot be recommended.

Simultaneous intrauterine pregnancy and an ectopic gestation is very rare but has been reported.

Delay in diagnosis still occurs in some 20% of cases with the diagnosis of a chronic ectopic still one of the most difficult to make.

Further reading

Confidential enquiry 1991–1993.

Macafee CAJ. Diagnoses not to be missed: ectopic pregnancy. *British Journal of Hospital Medicine*, 1982; **9**: 246–8.

Steer P. Surgery of ectopic pregnancy. In: Monaghan JM, ed. *Rob and Smith's Operative Surgery*, London: Butterworths, 1987; 248–54.

Yao M, Tulandi T. Current status of surgical and non-surgical management of ectopic pregnancy. *Fertility Sterility*, 1997; **67**: 421–33.

Related topics of interest

ENDOMETRIOSIS

This disorder is caused by the presence of functional ectopic endometrium. Its exact aetiology and pathogenesis is unknown.

Pathology

Endometriosis is a common disorder, especially in caucasian women, having a prevalence of 15–25% in most reported series. It is a disorder of the reproductive years, although post-menopausal endometriosis has been reported.

The most widely held theory is that of Sampson, who proposed the cause to be implantation of endometrial cells transported to the pelvic cavity by retrograde menstruation. Endometrial cells are also found in blood vessels and lymphatics and may embolize to distant sites.

Other theories are of coelomic metaplasia (Meyer) and transformation of embryonic cell rests.

Retrograde menstruation is an extremely common phenomenon as described at laparoscopy, and some unknown stimulus such as an autoimmune reaction may be necessary to establish endometriotic deposits.

Endometriotic implants are not identical to eutopic endometrium, having structural and functional differences which may be relevant in explaining the pathogenic effects.

There is an increased volume of free peritoneal fluid in the pelvis of women with endometriosis, and this fluid is rich in macrophages. Vasoactive amines released by macrophages may cause pelvic pain, and phagocytosis of sperm may be implicated in infertility associated with endometriosis.

The role of prostaglandins in inhibiting ovum release and interfering with tubal motility and the effect of increased concentration of prostaglandins associated with pelvic pain is unclear, with recent studies failing to confirm earlier theories.

Clinical features

The main symptoms are cyclical pelvic pain, deep dyspareunia and infertility. Cyclical bleeding from other organs may occur and rarely severe symptoms of intestinal obstruction or intraperitoneal bleeding.

Endometriosis is increasingly found as an incidental finding at laparoscopy, e.g. during laparoscopic tubal occlusion, and it is disputed that minimal endometriosis is implicated in pelvic pain and infertility, although success rates with assisted conception techniques are lower in the presence of minimal endometriosis.

Treatment

A wide range of medical treatment options are currently available. Success rates in improving symptoms, observing resolution of endometriotic deposits or achieving a successful pregnancy of the order of 60–80% have been reported in most published series. However, there is a high frequency of recurrent disease, of the order of 20% by 2 years.

Medical options include the synthetic steroid Danazol, the antiprogestagen Gestrinone, continuous progesterone therapy (e.g. medroxyprogesterone acetate) or GnRH agonist therapy, with or without concomitant HRT.

Non-steroidal anti-inflammatory drugs may have a role in controlling the pain of endometriosis.

Surgical options are radical or conservative conventional surgery and laparoscopic surgery, utilizing electrodiathermy or laser vaporization. The last treatment modality is reported to be very effective and safe, without the morbidity of open surgery and without the side-effects of medical therapy.

Further reading

Thomas EJ, Rock J. eds. *Modern Approaches to Endometriosis*. London: Kluwer, 1991.

Related topics of interest

FALLOPIAN TUBES

Normal tubal function is relatively easily disrupted because the delicate cilia are damaged, commonly by infection. Motility of the tube is important for normal function, and any pathological process causing the formation of pelvic adhesions can also impair tubal function.

Compromised tubes may become totally occluded, leading to infertility, or partially occluded, increasing the risk of tubal ectopic pregnancy.

Problems

1. *Infection.* Ascending pelvic infection causes oedema, which occludes the tube at its proximal and distal ends, forming a closed cavity that predisposes to cyst (hydrosalpinx) and abscess (pyosalpinx) formation.

Partial resolution of the infection leads to a chronic state in which the tubes are dilated and tortuous, with loss of functional cilia. The adjacent ovary may become involved, forming a chronic inflammatory tubo-ovarian mass.

Pelvic tuberculosis, although increasingly rare, invariably affects the tubes. Usually a secondary infection, the tubes are thickened and distended, with surrounding adhesions and granuloma formation. Caseation occurs within the lumen and ciliary function is lost. The tube often remains patent, with eversion at the fimbrial end.

2. *Malignant change.* Primary cancer of the Fallopian tube is extremely rare with an incidence of about 40 cases per annum in England and Wales. These are adenocarcinomata which may cause abnormal bleeding, in the form of a watery bloody vaginal loss, usually in post-menopausal women. Late presenting features are a pelvic or abdominal mass with ascites and evidence of metastatic spread, e.g. to the omentum, presenting and behaving in a similar manner to cancer of the ovary. Diagnosis is usually late and frequently unsuspected, even at laparotomy unilateral tubal enlargement is a suspicious feature.

3. *Endometriosis.* This may affect the tubes, either by direct involvement (some authorities maintain that this is unusual) or by adhesion to an adjacent (e.g. ovarian) focus.

Management

Prompt, effective antibiotic therapy is necessary to preserve tubal function.

Damaged tubes require laparoscopic assessment prior to reconstructive surgery in cases of infertility. Early ectopic pregnancy may be treated by evacuation and conservation of the tube if the latter is not severely damaged. Laparoscopic surgery is increasingly utilized to minimize post operative adhesion formation.

Persistent chronic infection with disabling pain and not controlled by long-term antibiotics requires pelvic clearance.

Tuberculosis is treated with chemotherapy, such as rifampicin, isoniazid and ethambutol. Treatment is effective and pelvic clearance rarely necessary.

Cancer of the Fallopian tube is staged at laparotomy in a similar manner to ovarian cancer.

Principles of treatment are identical, with optimal cytoreductive surgery followed by systemic chemotherapy using a platinum-based compound, alone or in combination.

Endometriosis causing a large tubo-ovarian mass is best treated by pelvic clearance. More conservative therapy is indicated if the patient wishes to preserve her fertility.

Further reading

Carty MJ. Pelvic tuberculosis. In: MacLean AB, ed. *Clinical Infection in Obstetrics and Gynaecology*. Oxford: Blackwell Scientific Publications, 1990: 255–61.

Lawton F, Lees C, Kelleher C. Primary cancer of the Fallopian tube. In: Studd J, ed. *Progress in Obstetrics and Gynaecology*, Vol. 12. Edinburgh: Churchill Livingstone, 1996: 393–402.

Shepherd JH. Cancer of the Fallopian tube. In: Shepherd JH, Monaghan JM, eds. *Clinical Gynaecological Oncology*, 2nd edn. Oxford: Blackwell Scientific Publications, 1990: 247–53.

Related topics of interest

FIBROIDS

Leiomyoma (fibroids) are the commonest tumours found in pre-menopausal women. Approximately 30% of women of reproductive age have fibroids, and in the USA they are the commonest indication for hysterectomy (approximately one third).

Problems

1. *Menorrhagia.* Submucus fibroids (30%).

2. *Infertility.* Impaired implantation.

3. *Pressure symptoms.* Urinary/bowel symptoms.

4. *Sarcomatous change.* 0.2% risk.

5. *Polycythemia.* Secretion erythropoetin like substance.

6. *Pelvic pain.* Degeneration or torsion.

Classification

1. *Submucous.* Project into the uterine cavity, can be polypoid, results in menorrhagia (~11%).

2. *Intramural.* Within the uterine wall, surrounded by a so called 'false capsule' (~73%).

3. *Subserous.* Seen on the surface of the uterus, can be pedunculated (~16%).

4. *Cervical.* Associated with delivery problems and surgical removal can be fraught.

5. *Intra-ligamentary.* Fibroid grows within broad ligament, cause ureteric compression.

6. *Parasitic.* A fibroid attached outside the uterus, i.e. the bladder.

Fibroids are composed of smooth muscle cells, arranged in whorls. Fibroids can undergo a variety of changes. Hyaline degeneration results in a more homogeneous consistency which in time can become cystic by liquefaction. Calcification can occur which enables X-ray diagnosis. Red degeneration in pregnancy results in localized pain and tenderness. Sarcomatous change is very rare (0.2%) but potentially fatal.

The aetiology of fibroids is unknown, although it is thought that there growth is dependant on oestrogen and progesterone as they appear to regress after the menopause, and HRT can stimulate growth. There is a 9-fold increase in fibroids in black women where they also occur at a younger age. The use of Depo-medroxy progesterone acetate and the combined oral contraceptive pill protects against developing fibroids.

Investigations

1.   Ultrasound scan. With expertise and the use of a vaginal probe it is possible to get an accuracy of approximately 80%. The difficulty arises when differentiation between a pedunculated fibroid and an ovarian mass becomes necessary.

2.   MRI. Allows for better differentiation between an ovarian mass and a fibroid uterus.

3.   Laparoscopy. Direct visualization can be important.

4.   Hysteroscopy. Important in assessment of infertility and recurrent miscarriage to detect submucus fibroids or any further intrauterine pathology.

Treatment

Medical treatment with GnRH analogues reduce size by 36–49% within 3 months. Further shrinkage may occur, but on cessation of treatment the baseline volume returns within 6 months. Shrinkage rates are variable – less success in obese women, and those with high oestradiol levels after 3 months.

GnRH analogues may allow shrinkage such that a vaginal hysterectomy can be performed. They reduce anaemia (with increased ferritin, haemoglobin and haematocrit concentrations) and therefore the need for transfusion. Reduced intraoperative blood loss has also been reported.

Successful reduction of fibroid volume does not occur if add-back therapy is commenced simultaneously, therefore it should be delayed for 3 months. Add-back has been used successfully to treat fibroids for up to 2 years.

The antiprogesterone mifepristone has also been shown to decrease uterine volume and blood flow similarly to GnRH.

Surgical treatment is classically by hysterectomy, usually by the abdominal route. A midline incision may be necessary. Fibroids should be treated if in excess of 12 weeks or symptomatic. Vaginal hysterectomy is advocated by some for fibroids up to 20 weeks.

Myomectomy is advocated in the young woman wishing to conserve her fertility, but the recurrence rate can be as high as 30%. The use of vasopressin has been advocated to reduce blood loss at myomectomy. Simultaneous hysterectomy is a significant risk and the patient must be warned of this.

Hysteroscopic removal with or without simultaneous endometrial ablation is an option. Pedunculated and submucus fibroids can be shaved to the level of the uterine cavity. For larger fibroids devascularization followed by removal as a two-stage procedure is advocated.

Laparoscopic myomectomy requires considerable skill and may be a lengthy operation. The upper limit of the fibroid is 10 mm and there should be no more than four present. Interstitial laser photocoagulation has also been successfully used, where the laser is inserted into the centre of the fibroid resulting in necrosis.

Further reading

Corscaden JA, Singh BP. Leiomyosarcoma of the uterus. *American Journal of Obstetrics and Gynecology*, 1958; **75:** 149–53.

Loeffler FE, Noble AD. Myomectomy at the Chelsea Hospital for women. *Journal of Obstetrics and Gynaecology of the British Commonwealth*, 1970; **77:** 167–70.

Sutton C. Treatment of large uterine fibroids. *British Journal of Obstetric Gynaecology*, 1996; **103:** 494–6.

West CP. LHRH analogues in the management of uterine fibroids, premenstrual syndrome and breast malignancies. *Bailliere's Clinical Obstetrics and Gynaecology*, 1988; **2:** 689–709.

Related topics of interest

FISTULAE IN OBSTETRICS AND GYNAECOLOGY

A fistula is defined as a communication between two epithelial or endothelial surfaces. It is usually an acquired condition. Vesico-vaginal fistula has four major causes:

- Surgical: Hysterectomy, LSCS.
- Obstetric: CPD, Forceps delivery.
- Radiotherapy: Vault caesium etc.
- Congenital.

The commonest cause of a vesico-vaginal fistula (V-V) is surgical misadventure, whereas in the third world it is obstructed labour.

If bladder damage is noted at the time of surgery then it should be repaired in two layers with plain cat gut, followed by 10–12 days free urinary drainage via a catheter so allowing the formation of a cicatrix.

Symptoms

Urinary leakage can give clues as to the site of the fistula. Total incontinence usually means a large V-V fistula. Continuous incontinence with voluntary micturition implies a ureterovaginal fistula. Frequency and urge incontinence can be due to a small V-V fistula.

The 3-swab test will determine the level of the fistula by which swab becomes stained with methylene blue that has been instilled into the bladder; direct vision of the fistula is better.

If a higher fistula is suspected then a micturating cystogram and IVU will be required to see the level of the fistula or the obstruction.

Management

Conservative management if small, requiring free catheter drainage for up to 12 weeks has been reported. Surgical repair can be performed immediately or as a planned procedure when 8 weeks should elapse between the time of damage and repair. The repair of a V-V fistula should be performed by an experienced surgeon as the chances of success are highest at the first attempt. There should be adequate exposure, careful dissection of the fistula, accurate suturing of the bladder in two layers without tension followed by closing the vagina so as to act as a double breast support. Secure catheter drainage (supra-pubic) is mandatory. Following surgery the repair is checked with methylene blue to confirm that it is water tight.

A low fistula is repaired via the vaginal route with the patient in the knee-chest position. In high fistula then a combined abdominal-vaginal procedure may be needed. The use of a Martius graft has been advocated (labia major) to support a low repair and occupies a position between the bladder neck and the vagina, in a similar way that omentum can be introduced when an abdominal procedure is performed.

The most difficult V-V fistula to repair are those after radiotherapy where the success rate is only 50%

Post-operatively it is important to have a good output of dilute urine. Free catheter drainage is essential to avoid retention and therefore put tension on the suture line. Prophylactic antibiotics are often considered.

Urinary tract

Damage to the ureters can occur during any abdominal or vaginal operation. Two-thirds of ureteric injuries occur during abdominal hysterectomy, compared to one-third for the vaginal route.

Transection will result in extravasation of urine followed by abdominal pain and likely infection as urine is extremely irritant. If noted at operation then reconstitution can occur over a stent using an absorbable suture and a drain placed at the site of the ureteric anastamosis. The stent should be left in for between 10–14 days and then removed via a cystoscope. Later repair is more difficult because of fibrosis. There are various techniques used for re-implantation of the ureter into the bladder. This can be done directly using an anti-reflux procedure. If the length is too short then the bladder can be brought up via a psoas hitch operation or by fashioning a Boari flap, so relieving the tension. If the ureter is still to short then a transuretero-ureterostomy can be performed.

Obstruction is treated by relieving the blockage; this can be performed from below using a stent, or may need resection or reimplantation.

Fistula between the ureter and the vagina will usually mean re-implantation of the ureter as described previously, although occasionally the insertion of a stent can evoke healing without major surgery.

Further reading

Brudnell M. Medico-legal aspects of ureteric damage during abdominal hysterectomy. *British Journal of Obstetrics and Gynaecology,* 1996; **103:** 1180–3.

Podratz KC. Vesicovaginal fistula. In: Monaghan JM, ed. *Rob and Smith's Operative Surgery.* 1987; 127–42.

Riddle PR. Surgery of the upper urinary tract. In: Kirk RM, Williamson RCN, eds. *General Surgical Operations.* Edinburgh: Churchill Livingstone, 1987; **14:** 222–38.

Sims JM. On the treatment of vesicovaginal fistula. *American Journal of Medical Sciences,* 1852; **23:** 59–82.

Related topics of interest

Abdominal versus vaginal hysterectomy (p. 1)
Forceps and ventouse (p. 215)

GENITAL PROLAPSE

This occurs predominantly in old age and rarely congenitally. It is a consequence of pelvic fascial relaxation associated with the reduction in hormone levels and parturition. It is particularly associated with multiparity, traumatic vaginal delivery, large babies, bearing down prior to full dilatation, prolonged second stage, poor nutrition and congenital weakness such as in spina bifida. Increased abdominal pressure due to obesity, chronic obstructive airways disease, smoking, chronic constipation, ascites and abdominal masses such as uterine or ovarian tumours are also associated with prolapse.

Grading prolapse

This is based on clinical examination and is divided into uterine descent and vaginal wall descent.

1. Uterine descent

- *First degree:* descent of the uterus within the vagina.
- *Second degree:* descent through the introitus on straining.
- *Third degree:* permanent descent through the introitus, commonly referred to as procidentia.

2. Vaginal wall descent

- *Urethrocele:* prolapse of the lower vagina.
- *Cystocele:* prolapse of the bladder base.
- *Enterocele:* hernia and prolapse of the pouch of Douglas.
- *Rectocele:* prolapse of the posterior vaginal wall.
- *Vault prolapse:* follows hysterectomy, can be associated with an enterocele (uncommon).

Presentation

The majority (80%) of patients present complaining of 'something coming down'. The degree of prolapse bears little relationship to the symptoms.

Symptoms include frequency of micturition, incomplete emptying of bladder and bowel necessitating digital pressure.

Back and abdominal pain is a rare presentation of prolapse.

Decubital ulceration will cause bleeding and discharge, often associated with a procidentia.

Coital difficulties can occur as a result of the alteration of the vaginal anatomy.

Treatment

1. Prevention. Shorter labours and decreased family size, along with improved general health, nutrition and the increased use of hormone replacement therapy at the menopause are all preventive.

Caesarean sections – some mothers are now requesting an elective Caesarean section to prevent this condition. Increased use of physiotherapy post-natally may also help.

The use of oestrogen creams for 2 weeks prior to surgery is helpful in improving the vaginal and cervical tissues.

2. Pessaries. Ring, shelf and cup and stem pessaries have all been used in the past, but are used less frequently now, and only for patients unable to undergo anaesthesia. Shelf ('Simpson') pessaries have recently been withdrawn because of problems with their coating.

A ring pessary may be used for the temporary relief of symptoms prior to surgery, or in the last weeks of pregnancy if the mother has prolapse resulting in urinary incontinence.

There are now very few patients who cannot be operated on using modern anaesthetic techniques, especially regional blockade. Pessaries can cause vaginal ulceration and bleeding, and can erode through into the rectum and urethra.

If a ring pessary is used it is important to combine it with an oestrogen cream, and it must be cleaned and replaced every 6 months.

3. Surgery. The definitive procedure for uterine prolapse is a vaginal hysterectomy, which, if necessary, can be combined with the appropriate repairs.

It is important when performing a vaginal hysterectomy to follow steps that will result in good vaginal vault support using the transverse cervical and utero-sacral ligaments. Obliteration of the space between the uterosacral ligaments is important by use of a suture to prevent enterocele formation.

Anterior and posterior colporrhaphy are used alone when anterior or posterior wall prolapse occurs without uterine prolapse.

If stress incontinence is present the combination with urethral buttress sutures should be used, although in cases of pure stress incontinence without prolapse then colposuspension is a better procedure.

A Manchester repair produces uterine elevation by approximating the shortened cardinal ligaments anterior to the cervix and suturing them to the cervical stump following its amputation; it is combined with an anterior colporrhaphy. It is the procedure of choice if the patient needs to retain the uterus for fertility.

Le Fort's operation is rarely performed. In this procedure apposition of the anterior and posterior vaginal walls occurs, allowing two narrow lateral canals to exist. It is used only for major degrees of prolapse and prohibits intercourse.

Post-hysterectomy vaginal prolapse is rare and is treated by an abdominal procedure of sacral colpopexy using a mesh or fascia. Trans-vaginal fixation to the sacro-spinous ligament has been reported, but this is a blind procedure and has risks of visceral damage. Even with expert surgery recurrence rates of up to 25% have been reported.

Vaginal packing is beneficial prior to definitive surgery for procidentia, thus returning the anatomy to normal and allowing ulceration (if present) to heal.

Further reading

Evans AS. Operations for genital prolapse. In: Monaghan JM, ed. *Rob and Smith's Operative Surgery*. London: Butterworths, 1987; 92–104.

Jackson S, Smith P. Diagnosing and managing genitourinary prolapse. *British Medical Journal*, 1997; **314:** 875–8.

Milton PJD. Utero-vaginal prolapse. In: Studd J, ed. *Progress in Obstetrics and Gynaecology*, Vol 7. Edinburgh: Churchill Livingstone, 1989; **21:** 319–30.

Related topics of interest

Anatomy of the female pelvis, the fetal skull and the fetal circulation (p. 166)
Urinary incontinence: incontinence and retention (p. 135)

GESTATIONAL TROPHOBLASTIC DISEASE

Gestational trophoblastic disease comprises those conditions in which abnormal proliferation (neoplasia) of trophoblastic tissue occurs. This ranges from the relatively benign hydatidiform mole to the highly malignant choriocarcinoma. Molar changes have been suggested to be an exaggerated reaction of trophoblastic tissue which normally invades adjacent myometrium and may embolize via blood vessels. Choriocarcinoma may be metastatic from an unsuspected placental primary malignancy.

Classification

Gestational trophoblastic disease is classified by its pathological features, divided into: complete and partial hydatidiform mole, invasive mole, gestational choriocarcinoma and placental site tumour.

Pathology

Hydatidiform mole shows hydropically dilated trophoblastic villi, forming vesicles, associated with small areas of normal trophoblast. The complete mole is formed from paternal genetic material, usually from 23X chromosomal material, duplicating to 46XX in 90% of cases.

The partial mole shows evidence of a fetus as part of the same conception and is therefore genetically distinct.

Invasive mole invades deep into the myometrium, beyond the usual depth of placental implantation. It is distinguished from frank choriocarcinoma by the presence of chorionic villi.

Choriocarcinoma is composed of trophoblast tissue with absent villi, being a haemorrhagic mass of cyto- and syncytiotrophoblast. It readily metastasizes, principally to adjacent pelvic organs, lungs and brain.

Clinical features

Diagnosis of this condition is facilitated by measurement of β HCG, which is produced in abundance by trophoblast cells. The measurement is useful as a tumour marker to monitor treatment and in early detection of recurrent disease.

The overall prevalence in the UK is 0.7–1.0 per 1000 pregnancies. In other areas of the world, notably in SE Asia, the incidence is much higher.

The risk of developing the disease is higher at the extremes of reproductive life, increasing six-fold before age 15 and 26-fold after age 45.

Other predisposing factors include blood groups (higher if partners have different A and B groups and if the mother is group B or AB). Women with a balanced genetic translocation are also at increased risk of developing the disease.

Presenting symptoms include exaggerated early pregnancy symptoms, notably nausea and vomiting; vaginal bleeding with the passing of vesicles may occur and the patient may notice a rapidly enlarging abdominal mass.

Metastatic disease may present with pelvic pain, abnormal vaginal or rectal bleeding, haemoptysis, dyspnoea or bizarre neurological symptoms.

Examination may reveal an enlarged uterus, in advance of dates, signs of metastases, related to the chest or brain, or rarely intra-abdominal haemorrhage, e.g. from liver metastases.

Management

Diagnosis by history and examination and confirmed by elevated levels of β HCG is followed by treatment. Suction evacuation is employed for hydatidiform mole followed by close monitoring of β HCG levels. Regular urine samples are sent to a supraregional laboratory. Most patients have their β HCG levels return to normal (42% within 56 days). The urine levels are checked at 2-weekly intervals, for 6 months if the fall is rapid, otherwise for 2 years when patients are advised against a further pregnancy. After this time a further β HCG estimation is taken after any subsequent pregnancy.

Invasive mole may require hysterectomy and subsequent monitoring of β HCG levels.

Management of choriocarcinoma is complex and takes place in specialist centres. The tumour is very sensitive to chemotherapy and the results of treatment are excellent.

Treatment regimens are divided into low, medium and high risk depending on prognostic factors such as age, interval from and features of the antecedent pregnancy, e.g. a mole, abortion or full-term delivery, the level of β HCG, the ABO blood group, the size of the largest tumour mass and the site and number of metastases. It is also important to know whether previous treatment has been given, and, if so, whether with single or multiple agents.

Treatment regimens are complex and are continually being modified, therefore only examples of chemotherapeutic agents commonly employed are given.

Single-agent therapy is employed in low-risk regimens. The drug of choice is methotrexate (always with folinic acid rescue), to which the majority of these tumours are highly sensitive.

Other agents to which the tumour is sensitive and which are employed in medium- and high-risk regimens include etoposide, hydroxyurea, mercaptopurine, actinomycin D, vincristine, cyclophosphamide and cis-platinum.

Response is monitored by β HCG's estimation, chest X-ray and CAT head and body scans as appropriate.

Surgical excision of metastases which are resistant to treatment can improve survival.

The results of treatment generally are excellent with 5-year survival figures in excess of 90% in low-risk patients and 74% even in those presenting with quite advanced disease (presentation with cerebral metastases carries a poor prognosis with 25% of deaths occurring within 2 weeks of starting treatment).

Future fertility rates are good, with 75% of those who desired further children having at least one live birth.

Further reading

Begent RHJ. Trophoblastic disease. In: Shepherd JH, Monaghan JM, eds. *Clinical Gynaecological Oncology*, 2nd edn. Oxford: Blackwell Scientific Publications, 1990; 299–332.

Fox H. Gestational trophoblastic disease: Neoplasia or pregnancy failure? *British Medical Journal*, 1997; **7091:** 1363.

Related topics of interest

Cancer in pregnancy (p. 182)
Uterine tumours (p. 142)

HIRSUTISM

Hirsutism is increased growth of hair in women in a distribution similar to that of a male and it may occur in association with an oily skin and acne. It is not synonymous with virilism (although it may present as a feature of a virilizing syndrome), which is caused by excessive androgen exposure resulting in more widespread stigmata of the male: receding hairline, deepened voice, increased male-type muscle mass and distribution, clitoromegaly and atrophy of the breasts. Hirsutism *per se* does not have pathological implications, whereas virilism does, given that it may be indicative of an underlying neoplastic process, e.g. an ovarian tumour. Hypertrichosis is an increase in hair growth over all of the body, but this is usually fine, resembling lanugo, and again it does not have pathological implications.

Diagnosis

History and examination. Use photographs if possible. It is important to ascertain the ovulatory status of the woman, as ovulating women in the main have a low potential for serious pathology.

Investigations depend on androgen and associated hormone assays. The main androgens measured are dehydroepiandrosterone (DHEA), dehydroepiandro-sterone sulphate (DHEAS), androstenedione (A) and testosterone (T). In the female, androgens come from either the ovary or the adrenal. Androgen production is subject to diurnal rhythm, linked to the production and metabolism of cortisol. There is much debate as to the final common source of excess androgens in hirsute women, but most authorities believe it to be ovarian in origin. The ovary is under luteinizing hormone (LH) control, so conditions such as polycystic ovarian syndrome (Stein-Leventhal) lead to elevated A and T levels with hirsutism. The adrenal androgen production is under adrenocorticotrophic hormone (ACTH) control, so in conditions such as congenital adrenal hyperplasia (CAH), in which there is an enzymatic pathway disturbance, e.g. 21-hydroxylase deficiency, excess androgens are produced, and hence virilization occurs.

The severity of the disorder depends on a balance between production and clearance, most hirsute women having both increased production and clearance rates, with sex hormone-binding globulin (SHBG) being the final arbiter as to whether the clinical syndrome is expressed or not.

SHBG is a hepatically produced (under oestrogen and thyroid control) beta-globulin buffer that mops up excess androgens in the normal woman, but whose production is altered in the excess androgen woman. For example androgens diminish the level of SHBG, leading to reduced buffering and hence greater clinical androgen expression.

All of the above hormones or their metabolites may be assayed, or stimulation and suppression tests used, e.g. dexamethasone suppression. Radiological techniques such as selective catheterization and computerized tomography (CT) are also used.

Benign causes

- Racial.
- Idiopathic.
- Physiological – puberty, pregnancy, menopause.
- Drugs – dilantin, diazoxide, steroids, danazol.
- Porphyria.
- Traumatic.
- CNS linked – multiple sclerosis, encephalitis.
- Familial.
- Miscellaneous.

Other causes

- Ovarian – polycystic, hyperthecosis, virilizing tumours.
- Thyroid disease.
- Acromegaly.
- Adrenal – carcinoma, hyperplasia.
- Psychological – anorexia nervosa.
- Cushing's syndrome.
- Turner's syndrome.

Treatment

Simple suppression of the ovarian axis using the oral contraceptive pill is usually beneficial, as this lowers LH levels and increases SBHG levels. The progestogenic component of the combined pill is a competitive inhibitor of androgens at the hair follicle level. Norgestrel is the least androgenic progestogen. The infertile woman with polycystic ovarian syndrome may wish to become pregnant, and in this case clomiphene citrate is indicated. However, this drug increases LH levels and may exacerbate the hirsutism.

Steroids, primarily dexamethasone, 0.75 mg/day, or prednisolone, 10 mg/day, may be used. The aldosterone antagonist and potassium-sparing loop diuretic, spironolactone, 25 mg/day, decreases T production and is a competitive antagonist with T at hair follicle level.

It should be used with caution in those with hepatic and renal impairment and is contraindicated in pophyria, one of the causes of benign hirsutism.

The antiandrogen, cyproterone acetate, 100 mg/day on days 5–14 of the cycle, in conjunction with ethinyl oestradiol, 0.5 mg/day on days 5–25, decreases androgen production and is useful at the hair follicle and skin gland level as it diminishes sebum production.

The older hirsute woman may benefit from bilateral oophorectomy.

Associated modalities of treatment include any and all of the mechanical ways of removing unwanted and excess hair, e.g. electrolysis. More recently the use of ruby laser therapy, in non Q-switched mode, may offer a safer and more effective means of hair removal. The red light energy from the ruby laser is absorbed by the pigment in the hair shaft and the melanosomes of the hair bulb. Treatment is only effective for those hairs in the growing (anagen) phase. All of these treatments are time consuming and expensive. The regimens described will give relief to the majority of women, but bear in mind factors such as racial and familial hirsutism that may always be refractory to treatment.

Further reading

Shearman RP. Hirsutism and virilism. In: Whitfield CR, ed. *Dewhurst's Textbook of Obstetrics and Gynaecology for Postgraduates,* 4th edn. Oxford: Blackwell Scientific Publications, 1988; 80–90.

Related topics of interest

HORMONE REPLACEMENT THERAPY

Hormone replacement therapy (HRT) is the generic term given to oestrogen therapy for pre-, peri- and post-menopausal women suffering from disturbances of oestrogen metabolism. It must be combined with a progestogen for the last 10–13 days of the cycle, where the uterus is still present, to prevent unopposed oestrogen-related endometrial hyperplasia and malignancy. In conventional HRT regimes this has the disadvantage of inducing withdrawal bleeds at regular intervals. It is not contraceptive.

Climacteric symptoms
- Vasomotor – hot flushes, sweats.
- Vaginitis and vaginal atrophy.
- Dyspareunia and loss of libido.
- Cystitis and urethritis.
- Psychological dysfunction – loss of concentration, sleep disturbance, headaches, mood swings, depression, loss of energy.
- Altered skin and hair – thin and dry.
- Loss of height and bone and joint pain.
- Irregular menstrual bleeding.

Routes of administration
- Oral.
- Transdermal.
- Implant.
- Transvaginal.

Oral preparations are subject to hepatic and gut first-pass metabolism. Transdermal and subcutaneous implants may more closely mirror endogenous hormone activity. Implants have been linked with tachyphylaxis in supraphysiological concentrations and they may be linked with prolonged endometrial stimulation.

When libido and energy loss are major factors, HRT may be combined with subcutaneous depots of testosterone.

Preparations

The choice of oestrogen is dependent upon the indications, risks, convenience and patient compliance. Vaginitis in post-menopausal women will initially respond to topical oestrogen, but continuation of such a regimen for longer than a few weeks will result in unopposed endometrial stimulation due to absorbed oestrogen. The oestrogens utilized include ethinyloestradiol, mestranol, oestradiol, oestriol and conjugated oestrogens. More recent preparations are available to the confirmed postmenopausal women with an intact uterus (>12 months of postmenopausal amenorrhoea) in the form of continuous combined oestrogen and progestogen. These result in a thinned out atrophic endometrium leading to a 'non-bleed HRT' for the majority. Alternatively there is at least one preparation available as a 3 month long period cycle, again reducing the bleed phase associated with such combined preparations. The gonadomimetic preparation, tibolone, combines oestrogenic and progestogenic activity with weak androgenic activity, is 'non-bleed' and can also be given continuously to the woman with an intact uterus without cyclical progestogens. It is the author's experience that if there is any abnormal bleeding or breakthrough bleeding on these preparations then referral for investigation of the endometrial and ovarian axes should be mandatory.

Duration of treatment

HRT should be given until at least the age of 50 years, and for up to 10 years post-menopausally before relative risk factors for major risks such as breast cancer become an issue.

Major benefits

(a) There is clear evidence that HRT improves the quality and duration of life in post-menopausal women.

(b) HRT is associated with a reduced incidence of osteoporosis-induced fractures of the wrist, vertebral bodies and neck of femur. The data clearly show that calcium supplements, if the daily calcium intake is optimum around 800 mg, and exercise, do not confer any added protection against bone loss, at any age.

(c) A reduced incidence of stroke and myocardial infarction is also a benefit. The evidence is less clear when HRT is given with a progestogen, as the progestogen may blunt the oestrogenic protection.

Major risks

(a) There is an increased risk of endometrial hyperplasia and malignancy in woman with an intact uterus taking unopposed HRT. This risk is ablated if cyclical progestogens are added to their regimen.

(b) There is an increased risk of benign and malignant breast disease in women on unopposed HRT regimens for >10 years after the age of 50 years. This risk is reduced substantially below a relative risk of 1.0 if combined oestrogen-progestogen regimens are used, i.e. HRT may be breast protective with combined regimens. The only real contraindication to HRT is a recent history of breast cancer. There is evidence to suggest that if a breast cancer develops in a woman on HRT, then prognosis is improved.

(c) Gall bladder disease is increased in women on HRT.

(d) Hypertension, varicose veins, previous thrombotic episodes, endometriosis and fibroids are no longer thought to be contraindications to HRT.

Further reading

Studd JWW, Baber R. The menopause. In: Shaw RW, Soutter WP, Stanton SL, eds. *Gynaecology*. Edinburgh: Churchill Livingstone, 1992: 341–54.

Related topics of interest

Contraception and sterilization (p. 22)
Menopause (p. 72)
Premenstrual syndrome (p. 111)

HYPERPROLACTINAEMIA

Prolactin is secreted by the lactotroph cells of the anterior pituitary gland. It is primarily controlled by inhibition from the hypothalamus by dopamine and to a lesser extent gama-amino butyric acid.

Sustained hyperprolactinaemia (>1000 mU/l) requires further evaluation.

Causes

- Pituitary adenoma (40–50% of patients).
- Primary hypothyroidism (5% due to excess of TRH).
- Pharmacological causes (2% due to drugs that inhibit dopamine).
- Chronic renal failure.
- Chronic hepatic failure.
- Tumours compressing the pituitary stalk (so called pseudoprolactinoma, so decreasing dopamine secretion.
- Ectopic prolactin production by tumours.
- Stress.
- Idiopathic causes (35%).

Pregnancy results in a high prolactin, as does the initial post-partum period especially if breast feeding is practised. If the mother doesn't breast feed, prolactin will return to normal within 10 days.

Symptoms

Symptoms include galactorrhoea (occurs in between 30–80%), abnormal menstruation (commonly secondary amenorrhoea), infertility, hirsuitism, loss of libido, headaches and visual field defects. Women with PCOD have a 9.2% chance of having hyperprolactinaemia.

Drugs can result in hyperprolactinaemia, e.g.

- Phenothiazines: chlorpromazine, prochlorperazine.
- Benzamides: metoclopramide.
- Cimetidine.
- Methyldopa.
- Reserpine.
- Opiates.

Investigations

Examination including the breasts, a pelvic examination and a full neurological assessment. The latter should include visual field assessment to determine any effects on the optic chiasm.

The majority of tumours are less than 10 mm in diameter, and are called microadenoma. Larger tumours are referred to as macroadenoma.

Radiological diagnosis is difficult for microadenoma. The changes resulting in erosion of the clinoid process and the sella turcica (double floor) are more pathognomonic for macroadenoma. The use of CT scans and MRI have been used with varying degrees of success for diagnosis of the microadenoma.

The blood level of prolactin should be >600 mU/l and in the case of a macroadenoma can be higher than 8000 mU/l. It is important to assess each patient's T_4, because of the common co-existence of hyperthyroidism.

The natural pathogenesis of microadenoma is unknown. Approximately one-third of cases will undergo spontaneous resolution. Prolactin levels should be checked yearly.

Treatment

When to treat:

1. Microprolactinomas: if symptomatic (e.g. menstrual disturbance, galactorrhoea).

2. Macroprolactinomas: all, because of risk of tumour expansion.

3. Normal scan, but young and amenorrhoeic: treat because of risk of bone mineral density loss. Women with hyperprolactinaemic amenorrhoea can lose up to 25% of their vertebral bone density.

Medical

1. Bromocriptine. This drug is a dopamine agonist; it normalizes prolactin in over 90% of patients. It is given as an 8 hourly tablet with food, its main side effects being postural hypotension, nausea, vomiting, dizziness, syncope, constipation and cold peripheries. The starting dose of 1.25 mg/day is increased slowly up to 5 mg/day (effective in 66% cases), but may be increased to a maximum of 30 mg/day.

Treatment is monitored by prolactin levels with the aim of achieving a level of 200 mU/l. On this treatment, 60% of patients will have return of their periods within

3 months, and those desiring pregnancy 50% will succeed in 2 months.

2. Carbergoline. This drug is a long acting oral dopamine agonist. It has fewer side effects than bromocriptine, but is equally as effective in reducing prolactin levels (90%) and preventing puerperal lactation.

The dose is 0.25 mg twice a week, increasing to 1 mg twice weekly as required.

It is effective in patients resistant to bromocriptine, but the lack of adequate safety data during pregnancy and the puerperium suggest caution.

3. Quinagolide. This drug again is a long acting dopamine agonist which is useful in patients who are resistant to bromocriptine and carbergoline, although the cost may be prohibitive.

Shrinkage of the tumour occurs rapidly although hormone levels may be slower to respond. Continual improvement occurs with prolonged treatment. Maintenance doses can be quite low, but should be continued indefinitely as tumour regrowth can occur after cessation. Once pregnancy has occurred the bromocriptine should be stopped and tumour enlargement monitored by visual field assessment. Expansion of the tumour does occur with 25% chance in a macroadenoma and 1–5% chance in a microadenoma.

Surgery

Surgical treatment has been advocated in the past with Trans-sphenoidal excision of the tumour, however there is a high recurrence rate, with approximately 90% with macro- and 40% with micro-adenomas.

Radiotherapy using the linear accelerator, cobalt, yttrium implant or a proton beam have all been advocated. However now both surgery and radiotherapy are only advocated for large tumours with suprasellar and frontal extension, and non-functioning macroadenomas with prolactin levels <3000 mU/l.

Further reading

Hull MGR, Abuzeid MIM. Amenorrhoea and oligomenorrhoea, and hypothalamic-pituitary dysfunction. In: Shaw RW *et al.* eds. *Gynaecology.* Edinburgh: Churchill Livingstone, 1992; **18:** 249–68.

Molitch ME. Management of prolactinomas. *Annual Reviews of Medicine*, 1989; **40:** 225–32.

Related topics of interest

Infertility – I (p. 57)
Infertility – II (p. 60)
Polycystic ovarian disease (PCOD) (p. 104)

INFERTILITY – I

Infertility affects 1:10 couples. *Primary* infertility are cases where there has been no previous pregnancy and *secondary* infertility are those where there has been a previous pregnancy, irrespective of its outcome.

Causes

- Anovulation: 21%
- Tubal factor: 14%
- Sexual dysfunction: 6%
- Endometriosis: 6%
- Mucus hostility: 3%
- Male factor: 24%
- Unexplained: 26%

History

It is important to assess both partners. Both must be asked about their previous medical, surgical (e.g. appendicectomy) and family history, about acquired STD and coital history.

Specific *female* questions concern previous pregnancies, menstrual history, hirsuitism, galactorrhoea, dyspareunia, contraception (e.g. IUCD) and conization/cautery.

Specific *male* questions concern mumps orchitis, occupation, testicular operations, drugs (e.g. alcohol, sulphasalazine) and sexual function.

Examination

It is important to confirm normal pelvic anatomy, and in the male, normal scrotal anatomy. Also, look carefully for signs of endocrine or other systemic diseases, hirsuitism, and tumours. The establishment of secondary sexual characteristics must be confirmed.

Investigations

1. Female

- Rubella titre (confirm immunity prior to treatment).
- Day 21 progesterone (>30 nmol/l suggest ovulation).
- FSH/LH – important to take at time of menses (irregular periods/anovulation).
- Prolactin (>800 mU/l associated with anovulation).
- Testosterone/androgens – if hirsute with erratic periods, may well have PCOD.
- Thyroid function tests.

- Basal body temperature charts (1°C rise at midcycle).
- Pelvic ultrasonography – PCOD, anovulation.

2. *Male*

- Semen analysis – should be performed after 3 days abstinence:

Blood tests are only performed in the male if there is an abnormality of a routine semen analysis (less than 10 million/ml).

Assessment

1.   Ovulation. The LH surge prior to ovulation can be detected by urinary kits (e.g. First response).

Ovulation is suggested by a mid-luteal progesterone level >30 nmol/l (Day 21 of a 28 day cycle). The luteinization of a follicle can be suggested by a rise in basal body temperature (progesterone is thermogenic). Progesterone will cause the oestrogenized endometrium to change from a proliferative to a secretory pattern, demonstrated histologically and morphometrically by an endometrial biopsy – luteal phase defects can also be excluded.

Follicular   tracking   with   transvaginal ultrasonography will also suggest ovulation. The dominant follicle will rupture and either disappear or become altered in appearance due to haemorrhage into the newly formed corpus luteum. The endometrium will thicken to 1 cm or above and change in pattern, losing its 'three lined appearance' that is visible prior to ovulation.

Biochemical assessment without ultrasonography will fail to detect luteinized unruptured follicles (LUF) that are reported to occur in 10% of cycles in infertile couples.

2.   Tubal factors. Tubal patency can be assessed by various methods. Hysterosalpingography (HSG) will outline the uterine cavity and tubes, but is hazardous because of radiological exposure.

HyCoSy (hysterosalpingo-contrast-sonography) employs transvaginal scanning. It is safe, and is as effective in assessing patent tubes as HSG. It offers the advantage of being able to visualize the ovaries and exclude fibroids and some other uterine abnormalities.

Laparoscopy and dye hydrotubation is the gold standard for assessing tubal patency. Although it involves a GA with its inherent risks, it does have the advantage of directly viewing the pelvic anatomy, and excluding pelvic pathology such as endometriosis, PID, PCOS and adhesions. It is much better than a hysterosalpingogram in this context. Tuboscopy and faloposcopy are still under evaluation.

Male factor infertility is extremely common. One of the most simple invasive investigations for this along with the semen analysis is the PCT which should be performed in the mid-cycle and within 150 minutes of intercourse. The couple should have abstained from intercourse for 3 days. It is then possible to assess cervical mucus, sperm motility and morphology. More complex tests such as the sperm penetration test, mucus hostility tests, a sperm swim up test are all regularly performed to assess abnormal sperm function.

The introduction of the hysteroscope has meant that visualization and potential treatment of intrauterine pathology is now possible. A formal D&C is now only indicated if significant endometrial pathology such as TB is suspected, because of complications may follow a D&C such as intrauterine adhesions. The use of endometrial sampling is now preferred.

Further reading

Moghissi KS, Wallach EE. Unexplained infertility. *Fertility and Sterility*, 1983; **39:** 5–21.

Thompson W, Heasley RN. Investigation of the infertile couple. In: Shaw RW *et al.*, eds. *Gynaecology*, 1992; **16:** 219–30.

Related topics of interest

INFERTILITY – II

The management of infertility can be divided into groups dependant on the underlying cause and will be discussed as such. Specific causes of infertility such as PCOS and hyperprolactinaemia will be discussed in the appropriate chapters.

Ovulation induction

This may be used alone or prior to intrauterine insemination or donor insemination.

1. Clomiphene citrate. Commercially available as a mixture of the *cis* and *trans* isomers which are a combination of a strong anti-oestrogen and a weak oestrogen. It works at the level of the hypothalamus by displacing oestrogen from hypothalamic receptor sites therefore removing negative feedback and thus increasing GnRH secretion.

Clomiphene should be administered from day 2 to day 6 of the cycle, at a dose of between 100 mg daily to a maximum of 150 mg/day. Occasionally, the use of mid-cycle hCG (5000 IU) is used to mimic the LH surge that may be absent.

Side effects include visual disturbances (yellow vision), hot flushes, vaginal dryness, breast tenderness, rashes and abdominal discomfort. Hyperstimulation does occur but is rare. Multiple pregnancy rates are reported to be about 6%. A total of 80% will ovulate and half will become pregnant.

If amenorrhoea/oligomenorrhoea occur, progestogen induced withdrawal can be used as a starting point for treatment.

Reasons for failure to conceive after successful ovulation induction include cervical mucus hostility, increased abortion rate and a detrimental effect on both endometrium and embryos.

Dexamethasone (high androgen levels) and bromocriptine (hyperprolactinaemia) can be added for resistant cases.

2. Tamoxifen. Similar to clomiphene (although not licensed) and used when the patient is unable to tolerate the former. The starting dose is 20 mg/day for 5 days, starting on day 2. Doses can be increased to 40 mg daily.

3. Cyclofenil. Not an anti-oestrogen, although research work is sparse. It is said to increase FSH levels and enhances production of thin watery mucus favouring sperm transport – a well recognized drawback of clomiphene.

4. Pulsatile GnRH. Administered in patients with hypogonadotrophic amenorrhoea.

5. Gonadotrophins. The first pregnancy using exogenous LH and FSH was reported in 1960.

Human menopausal gonadotrophin (hMG) is available in a number of preparations:

- Humegon and perganol contain FSH and LH in equal parts (75 IU).
- Normegon has a FSH:LH ratio of 3:1.

Dosage is 75 or 150 IU IM daily starting on day 2. Serial serum oestradiol and ultrasonography are used to monitor response. The dosage may need to be adjusted either up or down. Once there is a leading follicle greater than 20 mm diameter (no more than three >18 mm) then an injection of 5000 or 10 000 IU of hCG is administered, with advice to the patient to have intercourse over the next 36–72 hours. hCG (human chorionic gonadotrophin) is secreted by the placenta and obtained from the urine of pregnant females. It has the action of LH.

In patients with an inherently high level of LH (i.e. PCOD) the use of pure FSH has been advocated. There are a number of preparations:

- Urofollitrophin: FSH extracted from the urine of postmenopausal women (metrodin, orgafol).
- Follitrophin alpha: Recombinant FSH (gonal F or metrodin high purity).

Complications

1. Cyst formation. Functional, may be associated with high oestradiol levels and represent unruptured follicles.

2. Multiple pregnancy. Rates are increased in patients with PCOD by approximately 15–20%, the majority being twins. Transvaginal scans will help determine zygosity (number of follicles and sacs). The abortion rate (10–15%) and stillbirth rates (28%) are also quite high.

3. *Hyperstimulation (OHSS)*. Potential life-threatening complication, iatrogenic, can occur with any of the ovulation induction agents.

The syndrome is characterized by ovarian enlargement, fluid accumulation in the peritoneal, pleural and rarely pericardial cavities resulting in intravascular volume depletion and haemo-concentration.

It can be mild, moderate or severe (ovaries <8 cm, 8–12 cm, >12 cm diameter respectively). The incidence following standard ovulation induction regimes is 4%; this may increase to 8.4% when GnRH analogues have been used. The incidence of severe OHSS ranges from 0.25–0.9%. Where more than 30 oocytes are recovered the incidence is 23%. Oestradiol levels greater than 6000 pg/ml on the day of hCG injection are associated with a 38% risk. Both these factors increase the risk to 80%.

Other factors associated with OHSS:PCOD, >35 years old, conception cycles or exogenous hCG administration in the luteal phase.

Management

This should be supportive whilst waiting for the condition to resolve spontaneously. Aims are symptomatic relief, avoid haemoconcentration, prevent thromboembolism and maintain cardiorespiratory and renal function.

Investigations will include:

- USS (ovarian dimension, ascites, pleural effusion).
- Chest X-ray (CXR).
- HB and haematocrit.
- U&Es.
- Albumin and LFTs.
- Clotting screen.

Fluid replacement is important (DIC is rare), a CVP may be necessary.

Albumin >32 g/l + Hb <14 g/dl – crystalloid 3 litres/24 hours.

Albumin <30 g/l , Hb >16 g/dl or U >6 mmol/l – albumin 2 units + saline 2 litres/24 hours.

Potassium should be avoided because of the risk of hyperkalaemia.

Paracentesis and anticoagulation may also be necessary. If embryos are due to be replaced, they should be frozen and replaced at a later date.

Intrauterine insemination

This can occur in natural cycles once ovulation has occurred or in stimulated cycles accompanied by ovulation induction. The technique involves preparing the semen and injecting this through the cleansed cervix directly into the uterus. It is useful if there is endometriosis, sperm/mucus interaction or for cases of coital difficulty. Husband or donor sperm can be used. Success rates are good.

GIFT

Following ovarian stimulation to produce multiple follicles with gonadotrophins, hCG (5000 IU IM) is given when there are three or more follicles >18 mm diameter. 36 hours later transvaginal (or laparoscopic) egg recovery is performed often under sedation. The eggs are identified by the embryologist and then some (no more than 3) are mixed with the prepared semen and placed into the Fallopian tube.

Success rates of 28% have been reported. There is significant risk of an ectopic pregnancy. Excess oocytes can be fertilized *in vitro* and the embryos frozen, only the later procedure is licensed by the HFEA.

IVF

This involves the same process as for GIFT except that all of the oocytes are mixed with the prepared semen and observed for fertilization after 24 hours. A maximum of three embryos are then replaced after 36 hours directly into the uterine cavity. Success rates vary, the best are achieved in large units and are about 20–30%.

ICSI and microsurgical techniques

Ovulation and egg recovery are identical to IVF. ICSI involves the microscopic injection of one sperm (or more recently spermatid) directly into the cytoplasm of the oocyte. It is useful for couples with failed fertilization following IVF, and if there are antisperm antibodies or oligospermia.

High success rates (30% clinical pregnancy rate per treatment cycle) have been achieved. This will reduce the demand for donor sperm.

Spermatids may be obtained by microsurgical epididymal sperm aspiration (MESA), first described in 1984. Combined with ICSI fertilization rates are good (45–67% compared to 7% with conventional IVF).

If no epididymal sperm is available, testicular sperm extraction (TESE) can be performed, and this is then combined with ICSI. Fertilization rates may be lower (50%) but implantation rates are the same as for MESA-ICSI.

Donor eggs These are recovered by conventional techniques and then used in couples where there is premature menopause or conditions such as Turner's syndrome.

Further reading

Amso NN, Shaw RW. New frontiers in assisted reproduction. In: Shaw RW *et al.,* eds. *Gynaecology,* 1992; **17:** 231–48.

Edwards RG. *Conception in the human female.* 1980: Academic Press, London.

Gemzell CA *et al.* Human pituitary FSH. I. Clinical effect of a partially purified preparation. *Ciba Foundation Colloquia on Endocrinology,* 1960; **13:** 191–5.

RCOG Guidelines 2. Use of gonadotrophic hormone preparations for ovulation induction. 1994.

Related topics of interest

Hyperprolactinaemia (p. 53)
Infertility – I (p. 57)
Polycystic ovarian disease (PCOD) (p. 104)
Therapeutic abortion and the Human Fertilization and Embryology Act 1990 (p. 132)

INTERMENSTRUAL, POST-COITAL AND POST-MENOPAUSAL BLEEDING

Abnormal uterine bleeding that is not related to the menstrual period is a common and usually innocent symptom. However, cancers of the uterus, both of the cervix and of the corpus uteri, commonly present with one or other of these symptoms, and consequently the main principle of management must be to exclude a carcinoma as a possible cause of the presenting symptom(s). Assessment should proceed in a logical manner, based on the patient's age, hormone status and general health.

History

Relevant features of the history are:
(a) The time interval from the onset of symptoms to presentation, the frequency and amount of bleeding.
(b) The period of amenorrhoea if post-menopausal, as this is related to an increased incidence of carcinoma of the corpus uteri.
(c) Exogenous hormone therapy, e.g. oral contraception or hormone replacement therapy.
(d) There is often vaginal discharge associated with secondary infection of a cervical ectropion or carcinoma.
(e) Rarely there may be a history of a bleeding disorder or of trauma.

Examination

General physical examination is performed, noting the patient's fitness for general anaesthesia and signs of metastatic cancer, e.g. left supraclavicular lymphadenopathy.

Pelvic examination begins with inspection of the cervix, with smear and biopsy as indicated. Colposcopy may be required. Atrophic change is noted if present. Bimanual examination provides an assessment of the uterus and adnexae followed by a rectal examination if there is suspicion of malignancy.

Investigation

Investigations are performed as indicated and may include:
(a) Cervical smear, mandatory in all suspicious cases, and in the absence of a recent negative result.
(b) Vaginal or endocervical swab in the presence of a discharge.
(c) Punch biopsy of the cervix, preferably colposcopically directed.

(d) Trans vaginal ultrasonography to measure endometrial thickness (normally <5 mm in post-menopausal women).

(e) Aspiration cytology or histology of the uterine cavity.

(f) Hysteroscopy under local anaesthesia.

(g) Examination under anaesthesia, D&C with hysteroscopy.

Conclusion

Most women presenting with abnormal uterine bleeding will not have serious underlying pathology. The possibility of a malignant neoplastic cause will increase with age. It is mandatory to exclude malignancy prior to treatment, e.g. by cautery to the cervix or exogenous hormone therapy.

Cancer of the cervix does occur in young women and must be excluded in all patients, particularly during and shortly after pregnancy.

For persistent unexplained symptoms a rare cause such as carcinoma of the Fallopian tube must be considered.

Atrophic change to the lower genital tract is the commonest cause of post-menopausal bleeding. Further bleeding after an interval of over 6 months warrants reinvestigation in case of dual pathology.

Related topics of interest

Cancer of the cervix (p. 16)
Fallopian tubes (p. 33)
Premalignant disease of the cervix (p. 108)
Uterine tumours (p. 142)
Vaginal discharge (p. 145)

MALE SUBFERTILITY

In a third of cases of infertility the problem lies with the male partner, and in a further third there are problems in both partners or the infertility is unexplained.

Investigation

Investigation of the infertile couple involves simultaneous investigation of both partners, with the least invasive investigations as a first line.

In the male a thorough history will exclude coital problems and impotence, although these patients usually present to other clinics. Retrograde ejaculation may be a problem after surgery on the lower urinary tract.

Examination of the genitalia may reveal the presence of a varicocele or undescended or abnormally small testes, and rectal examination is performed to exclude tenderness of the prostate or seminal vesicles, suggestive of infection.

The standard test is semen analysis. A fresh semen sample is examined under the microscope and a mixed agglutination reaction is performed to exclude the presence of anti-sperm antibodies.

Normal ranges for semen analysis vary between laboratories, for example:

Volume: 2–5 ml per ejaculate
Number: 20–100 million/ml
Motility: >50% motile
Morphology: <50% abnormal forms.

Serum estimation of gonadotrophin levels and prolactin may be performed at the initial consultation or as a result of the semen analysis.

Second-line investigations may involve surgical exploration of the scrotum with open testicular biopsy and on-table vasography.

Treatment

Commonly the semen analysis may reveal oligozoospermia of no definite cause (usually defined as <20 million per ml).

Conservative treatment including stopping smoking, decreasing alcohol intake and wearing loose-fitting underclothes may effect a significant improvement. Some advocate cold douching of the testes.

Hormonal abnormalities are usually refractory to treatment, apart from hyperprolactinaemia (which usually presents as impotence) and the rare isolated FSH deficiency. Tamoxifen or clomiphene may be given on an empirical basis, although results are poor.

High-dose steroids have been given to men with anti-sperm antibodies, with some successful pregnancies, although there is a 6% frequency of serious side-effects such as necrosis of the femoral head.

Surgical treatment to correct a varicocele is occasionally employed, again with variable results.

Bypass of a blocked vas deferens is very successful in reversing vasectomy in the absence of antibodies, but, if there is an infective aetiology, such as tuberculosis, then surgical correction is much more difficult.

Maldescended testes should be recognized and treated in childhood, but occasionally such patients are seen in the infertility clinic. Small ectopic testes should be excised owing to the risk of malignant change, but reasonable-sized or solitary ectopic testes should be fixed. Return of spermatogenesis has rarely been reported in such patients.

Bladder neck repair is a difficult surgical procedure, and such patients should be referred to a centre with the appropriate expertise.

Semen manipulation

With the advent of IVF, the techniques employed in sperm preparation have been utilized for the benefit of oligospermic men, with counts as low as 0.5 million per ml giving suitable prepared samples. Split ejaculates are obtained, with the first, sperm-rich, fraction subjected to centrifugation and purification such that a sample of prepared sperm is used in IVF. A suitable sample may contain as few as 50 000 spermatozoa per ml. Figures for oocytes fertilized and successful implantation of those embryos as high as 56% and 75% respectively have been reported.

The advent of intracytoplasmic sperm injection (ICSI) has improved the outlook for oligospermic men; both secondary to occlusion or congenital absence of the vasa deferentia and non-obstructive causes e.g. germ cell hypoplasia. Sperm may be obtained from the epididymis or testis itself by open surgical or transcutaneous aspiration.

Further reading

Hewitt J, Cohen J, Steptoe P. Male infertility and *in vitro* fertilisation. In: Studd J, ed. *Progress in Obstetrics and Gynaecology*, Vol. 6. Edinburgh: Churchill Livingstone, 1987: 253–75.

Pryor JP. Treatment of male infertility. In: Studd J, ed. *Progress in Obstetrics and Gynaecology*, Vol. 3. Edinburgh: Churchill Livingstone, 1983: 334–45.

Vandervorst M, Tournaye H, Devroey P. Surgical recovery of sperm for intracytoplasmic sperm injection. In: Studd J, ed. *The Yearbook of the Royal College of Obstetricians and Gynaecologists 1996.* London: RCOG Press, 1996; 167–77.

Related topics of interest

MENARCHE

The menarche, which is the time of the first period, occurs during puberty. It is a time of immense physiological and psychological change, based on somatic growth spurts, gonadal and sexual characteristic development, set against a background of race, genetics, nutrition and environmental factors.

Precipitating factors

Hypothalamic neuroendocrine maturation leading to pulsatile gonadotrophin-releasing hormone (GnRH) production from the hypothalamus modulates gonadotrophin (FSH and LH) release from the pituitary, and this in turn releases gonadal sex steroids, secondary to an elevation in the hypothalamic threshold of sensitivity to circulating sex steroids. The sex steroids, e.g. oestradiol, cause action at specific endpoint receptors, leading to pubertal changes and menstruation.

Pubertal stages

Five stages are described:

P_1 Prepubertal.

P_2 Early breast budding, some axillary and pubic hair.

P_3 Increase in breast tissue, more and darker pubic hair, characteristic body odour.

P_4 Further breast tissue, adult pubic hair, acne with or without menarche.

P_5 Adult breasts and sexual hair, menarche.

P_2 occurs at a mean age of 10.5 years (range 9–12 years) and the pubertal growth spurt occurs occurs between 11 and 14.5 years. Girls reach their final height within 3-4 years of the onset of puberty, with complete epiphyseal fusion about 2 years after menarche.

Abnormal puberty

Puberty may occur early (precocious) or be delayed. Precocious puberty is defined as any secondary sexual characteristics occurring before the age of 8 years. Precocious puberty may be complete, incomplete (dissociated) or pseudo-precocious. Delayed puberty occurs when there are no signs of breast tissue or pubic hair by the age of 14 years. It may be constitutional, secondary to chronic malnutrition or systemic disease or gonadal insufficiency – primary or secondary. Abnormal puberty needs specialized investigations, diagnosis and treatment as it may be sinister, e.g.

ovarian oestrogen-producing tumours in pseudo-precocious puberty.

Further reading

Ducharme JR. Puberty: physiology and pathophysiology in girls. In: Studd J, ed. *Progress in Obstetrics and Gynaecology*, Vol. 5. Edinburgh: Churchill Livingstone, 1985: 195–221.

Related topics of interest

Menopause (p. 72)
Menstrual cycle physiology (p. 81)
Paediatric gynaecology (p. 93)

MENOPAUSE

The menopause is defined as the last menstrual period of a woman's life. This single event characterizes a number of significant changes, collectively known as the climacteric, or menopausal syndrome. The changes are primarily due to oestrogen deprivation consequent upon ovarian failure.

Events in the climacteric

1. *Vasomotor instability.* Hot flushes and night sweats are seen in 50–75%, and may last for 5 years in 25%.

2. *Genital atrophy.* This is seen in the vulva, vagina, cervix, uterus, ovaries, bladder, urethra, and supporting ligaments, leading to infection, dyspareunia, apareunia, frequency, dysuria and urgency.

3. *Skin and hair.* The skin thins and is prone to superficial laceration and bruising. The axillary and pubic hair are slowly lost and the head hair thins. There may be an increase in facial hair.

4. *Psychological.* Anxiety, forgetfulness, low self-esteem, loss of confidence, difficulty in concentration.

5. *Osteoporosis.* This is caused by an increase in bone resorption and relative loss of trabecular bone. May be due to an increased skeletal sensitivity to the actions of bone resorbing hormones. Results in significant rise in the incidence of femoral neck, vertebral body and wrist fractures, with consequent associated losses of mobility, rises in hospitalization costs and fracture-related deaths.

6. *Cardiovascular.* Plasma cholesterol, triglycerides and very low-density lipoproteins (VLDL) all rise, and high-density lipoproteins (HDL) fall. This results in an increase in ischaemic heart disease in the post-menopausal female cohort.

Diagnosis

The diagnosis is relatively simple when symptoms are clear cut. It may be aided by plasma FSH (high) and oestradiol (low) levels. Ensure that psychological symptoms are not caused by other life events. Phaeochromocytoma, carcinoid syndrome and thyroid disease may mimic the climacteric.

Treatment

Treatment significantly reduces the risks of fractures, genital atrophy and psychological symptoms. Mortality from fractures and ischaemic heart disease can be avoided. See HRT.

1. Non-hormonal. Non-hormonal treatment is mostly of little use. Clonidine may be beneficial in the treatment of symptomatic hot flushes.

2. Oestrogens. Now widely used and proved to be of value. Can be given orally, transdermally, vaginally or as a subcutaneous implant. Oral administration has the disadvantages that hepatic metabolism causes a significant inactivation of much of the oestrogen (the 'first-pass effect'); it may cause an increase in renin substrate production (especially dangerous in hypertensive patients); and it may cause an increase in thrombembolic disease in those with a positive history. Subcutaneous oestrogen produces plasma oestrogen profiles most closely mimicking those of an ovulatory cycle. The addition of subcutaneous testosterone may relieve psychosexual problems such as loss of libido.

3. Progestogens. There is an increasing use of these preparations on their own without oestrogens. The data are not yet available as their true efficacy and, despite the claims of many commercial preparations, their use should be resisted until they are fully evaluated.

There is a substantial body of evidence to show that vasomotor and psychological symptoms benefit from oestrogen replacement therapy, although the data are somewhat conflicting, as not all authors agree upon the psychiatric assessment. The literature is conclusive that oestrogens conserve bone mass in osteoporotic and non-osteoporotic women, but that osteoporosis is not reversible. Oestrogen is demonstrably superior to calcium, sodium fluoride, vitamin D and thiazide diuretic therapy in this regard.

Hazards

The incidence of thromboembolic disease is not increased by natural oestrogen in post-menopausal women with no previous history. Natural oestrogen treatment does not adversely affect the cardiovascular system. There are some data to show that oestrogen treatment may be linked with breast cancer, but a relative risk >1.0 does not occur until some years after commencement of treatment. Unopposed oestrogen therapy in the post-menopausal woman with a uterus is associated with endometrial hyperplasia and frank malignancy, and this association is positively correlated with dose and duration. For this reason combined oestrogen-progestogen therapy (leading to a monthly withdrawal bleed, or three monthly withdrawal bleeds or 'non-bleed' cycles) is recommended in such women. Such a combination is less effective in preventing symptoms, especially psychological, than oestrogen alone, and may be linked to an increase in thromboembolic disease.

Further reading

Whitehead, MI. The climacteric. In: Studd J, ed. *Progress in Obstetrics and Gynaecology*, Vol. 5. Edinburgh: Churchill Livingstone, 1985; 332–61.

Related topics of interest

Contraception and sterilization (p. 22)
Hormone replacement therapy (p. 50)
Menarche (p. 70)

MENORRHAGIA – I

Menorrhagia is defined as excessive regular menstrual bleeding; objectively it is a blood loss in excess of 80 ml. It is a very common complaint, with about 30% of women between the age of 16 and 45 years suffering from menorrhagia. Of those, 5% will consult their GPs, and the complaint accounts for 15% of gynaecological referrals. It is the commonest indication for a hysterectomy. Menstrual blood loss shows a skewed distribution with a mean of 35 ml and a 90th centile of 80 ml. A total of 90% of the menstrual blood loss occurs within the first 3 days. Measurement is by the alkaline haematin method.

Aetiology

In 50% of women with proven menorrhagia no pathology is found at hysterectomy. In the remaining the causes are:

1. Local pelvic pathology

- Fibroids.
- Endometriosis.
- Pelvic inflammatory disease.
- Endometrial polyps.
- Carcinoma of uterine body/cervix/ovary.

2. General medical causes

- Hypothyroidism/hyperthyroidism.
- Coagulation disorders: Von-Willebrand's/ITP.

3. Iatrogenic causes

- Intrauterine contraceptive devices.
- Progesterone only contraception.
- Anticoagulant therapy.

Management

Treatment should be directed to the cause. However as over 50% of patients have no demonstrable cause (dysfunctional uterine bleeding – DUB) for their menorrhagia, the majority of treatment has to be empirical. The use of endometrial biopsy techniques prior to treatment is widespread, especially the use of the outpatient endometrial sampling. Menorrhagia can cause iron deficiency anaemia which often requires iron therapy.

Drug therapy

1. Antifibrinolytic agents. Tranexamic acid is used on the premise that fibrinolytic action is abnormal in menorrhagia. The dosage is 1–1.5 g qid during menstruation. Side-effects of thromboembolism means that women with previous history of thrombosis or low levels of antithrombin III should not receive it. It reduces blood loss by 54%.

2. Prostaglandin synthetase inhibitor. Mefenamic acid is the most commonly used; it reduces the menstrual blood loss by an average of 20–30%. It only need be taken during menstruation. The effectiveness is due to the excessive levels of uterine prostaglandins. The dosage is up to 500 mg qid during menstruation. Few side-effects, but contraindicated in women who suffer from peptic ulceration.

3. Ethamsylate. This is thought to increase capillary wall strength and can reduce menstrual blood loss, but it is not as effective as tranexamic acid.

4. Progestogens. The use of progestogens was based on the theory that women with menorrhagia have anovular cycles, however this is unsubstantiated.

Progestogens are more useful in regulating menstrual cycles, although up to 30 mg of norethisterone daily will usually stop vaginal bleeding within 48 hours.

The usual dosage of norethisterone is 15 mg from days 15–27.

5. Oral contraceptives. Often used in the young patient when contraception is often required.

6. Danazol. A testosterone derivative, acts on the hypothalamic pituitary ovarian axis, as well as directly on the endometrium. Inhibits ovulation but is not contraceptive.

The dosage is 200–800 mg daily for up to 6 months. Side effects are androgenic causing acne, hirsuitism and weight gain. Permanent voice change can occur.

7. Gestrinone. This is a synthetic trienic 19-norsteroid with antigonadotrophic and antiprogesterone activity. It is claimed to have much fewer side effects than danazol. The usual dose is 2.5 mg twice weekly.

8. GnRH analogues. These induce a medical menopause. They are effective if used alone, but the induced hypoestrogenic state causes a reduction in bone density. Administered with cyclical HRT, they reduce the duration of menses and number of days of heavy loss. They are very expensive. They can be administered as a nasal spray (Buserelin), as a depot injection (Goserelin) or a subcutaneous bolus injection (Leuproline).

9. HRT. Often used around the period of the climacteric. It has been reported to be clinically successful in menopausal women with menorrhagia.

Further reading

Bonnar J, Sheppard BL. Treatment of menorrhagia during menstruation: randomised control trial of ethammsylate, mefenamic acid and tranexamic acid. *British Medical Journal,* 1996; **313:** 579–82.
Cameron IT. Dysfunctional uterine bleeding. *Clinical Obstetrics and Gynaecology,* 1989; **3:** 322–4.
Higham JM. Medical treatment of menorrhagia. In: Studd J. ed. *Progress in Obstetrics and Gynaecology,* Vol. 9. Edinburgh: Churchill Livingstone, 1991; **21:** 335–48.

Related topics of interest

Menorrhagia – II (p. 78)
Minimally invasive surgery (p. 84)

MENORRHAGIA – II

After medical treatment, between 20 and 40% of patients will require some form of surgical intervention. In 1985 no fewer than 18 600 hysterectomies were performed for purely menstrual disorders. In 1988 new endometrial ablative techniques were introduced.

The aim of both endometrial ablation and resection is to remove the part of the uterus that bleeds abnormally and allow the lining of the uterus to become lined with a layer of fibrous tissue. The fact that intrauterine adhesions resulted in amenorrhoea or at least a reduction of menstrual flow was first reported by Asherman in 1948.

Techniques of ablation
- Cryocoagulation.
- Laser ablation (ELA).
- Endometrial resection (TCRE).
- Radiofrequency ablation (RAFEA).

Endometrial resection

This procedure was first described by Neuwirth for resection of submucus fibroids. It was De Cherney who first used the technique for intractable menstrual bleeding.

Endometrial resection was introduced into the UK in Oxford in 1988. It is performed under direct vision and takes approximately 20–30 minutes to perform. It can be performed as a day case.

The uterine cavity needs to be distended and irrigated. Glycine 1.5% is the distension medium of choice.

Patient selection is very important, based on the following criteria:

- Purely menorrhagia.
- Uterus size < 10 weeks.
- Proliferative phase or pretreatment.
- More effective for older patients.
- No endometriosis/adenomyosis.
- Family complete (although not contraceptive).
- Gravid (procedure often extremely difficult in nuliparae).

Complications of perforation, haemorrhage and fluid overload (dilutional hyponatraemia, cf. TURP syndrome), gas embolism and also infection have been reported.

Laser ablation

This technique was first described by Goldrath. A Nd-Yag laser is used for photovapourization of the endometrium. The endometrium is destroyed to a depth of 5 mm.

There are three techniques: *touch, non-touch, combination*. The whole of the endometrial cavity is treated, taking approximately 45–50 minutes. It is also performed under direct vision using glycine as the distension medium.

Post operatively a bloody and sero-sanguinous vaginal discharge can occur for up to a month.

The procedure can be repeated as there is a shallow learning curve.

Theoretically there may be a lower risk of perforation with this technique, but there appears to be a higher rate of fluid overload as well as more risks to the theatre staff.

Poor results are associated with young patients, fibroids, enlarged uterine cavity >10 cm and adenomyosis.

Success rates

Preliminary evidence from the RCOG mistletoe study shows a commulative failure rate for TCRE of 18% and for ELA of 32%.

Patient satisfaction was 74% for TCRE and 64% for ELA.

Radiofrequency-induced thermal ablation

This is a blind technique described by Phipps. It requires no surgical training and relies on heating the endometrium to cytotoxic levels by means of radiofrequency electromagnetic thermal energy, which is delivered by a probe placed inside the uterine cavity.

It can be performed as a day case and takes about 20 minutes. The overall menstrual improvement is seen in approximately 80% of patients.

The manufacturer recommends that RAFEA is only suitable for a regular uterus, excluding many patients, and necessitating preoperative hysteroscopy.

Risks of vesicovaginal fistulae are present if the vagina is not totally protected from thermal energy.

If perforation occurs, the potential for thermal necrosis of the intra-abdominal contents is a real risk.

There has recently seen the introduction of thermal balloon techniques which may in time be a further option.

Discussion

Preparation of the endometrium (TCRE and ELA) with thinning agents is advised, if the operation cannot be performed during or immediately after menstruation. Atrophic endometrium reduces operating times and increases success rates but does not significantly decrease complication rates. GnRH analogues and Danazol are effective choices when given for 6–8 weeks beforehand. Progestogens are less successful.

It would appear that laser ablation and endometrial resection have similar success rates, but that radiofrequency ablation has now fallen out of favour. TCRE may be quicker and cheaper. Laser treatment seems to be safer. Resection alone (without rollerball diathermy) has significantly greater complication rates.

It is however still early days for all these treatments, and long-term follow-up is essential to rule out any late complications.

All the new techniques are patient friendly, associated with a much shorter stay in hospital, faster recovery and much cheaper. Even if these techniques are unsuccessful, the recourse to hysterectomy is available. With this in mind it is imperative when the patient is asleep to assess suitability for a vaginal hysterectomy.

Subsequent pregnancies have been reported, hence contraceptive advice is essential. Hormone replacement therapy is not contraindicated but must be a combined preparation.

Further reading

Goldrath MH, Fuller TA, Segal S. Laser photovapourization of endometrium for the treatment of menorrhagia. *American Journal of Obstetrics and Gynaecology,* 1981; **140:** 14–19.

Magos AL, Baumann R, Turnbull AC. Transcervical resection of the endometrium in women with menorrhagia. *British Medical Journal,* 1989; **96:** 1209–12.

Parkin DE. Laser ablation or endometrial resection. In: Studd J, ed. *Progress in Obstetrics and Gynaecology,* Vol. 12. Edinburgh: Churchill Livingstone, 1996; 345–54.

Phipps JH, Lewis BV, Roberts T *et al.* Treatment of functional menorrhagia by radiofrequency-induced thermal endometrial ablation. *Lancet,* 1990; **335:** 374–6.

Related topics of interest

MENSTRUAL CYCLE PHYSIOLOGY

There is little ovarian follicular development in childhood; what there is results in atresia. Full follicular development is only possible with hypothalamic–pituitary–ovarian axis maturation at puberty. Once maturation has commenced follicles proceed to either ovulation or atresia, the fate of the majority. At menarche each ovary contains about 500 000 primordial follicles, each consisting of an oocyte, arrested in meiotic prophase, surrounded by granulosa cells and a membrane, the basal lamina, separating the follicle from surrounding stroma. Oocyte-granulosa communication occurs via the cytoplasmic processes to provide nutrients and possibly facilitating inhibition of oocyte maturation.

Follicular development

A primordial follicle proliferates to a multilaminar primary follicle with a central enlarged oocyte surrounded by the zona pellucida and then the stratum granulosum covered by the two theca layers, interna and externa. Granulosa cells coalesce, forming follicular fluid and an antrum in the Graafian follicle. The antrum further enlarges and divides the granulosa cells into the membranum granulosum and the cumulus oophorus. Immediately prior to ovulation the follicle consists of an innermost secondary oocyte with the first polar body, surrounded successively by the zona pellucida, the corona radiata and the cumulus oophorus. After ovulation the granulosa and theca cells form the gonadotrophic and luteotrophic corpus luteum (hence the rationale behind luteal phase support in some pregnancies when it is felt to be deficient), which degenerates to form a corpus albicans if no pregnancy occurs. Primordial to antral phase development takes 85 days, resulting in a follicle of 2–5 mm diameter, with subsequent growth being 1–3 mm/day, so that at the time of the LH surge and ovulation a dominant follicle measures 20±3 mm. Each dominant follicle is usually surrounded by 2–3 non-dominant ones measuring <16 mm, and they are not generally released at ovulation.

Endometrial development

Immediately after menstruation the endometrium is resurfaced, leading to small, short, tubular, ovoid, basally or centrally nucleated epithelial glands that are columnar or cuboidal. The glands and surrounding stroma show increased mitoses, with elongation, tortuosity and columnar shape by late follicular phase.

The early follicular phase rise in FSH primes granulosa cells in the maturing follicle to produce oestradiol via aromatase enzyme induction. LH receptors then appear on granulosa cells, and this appearance is enough to maintain aromatase activity (and hence oestradiol production) as FSH declines in the follicular phase. The rising oestradiol feeds back to the pituitary and causes an LH surge mid-cycle and a lesser FSH surge. There is then a sharp decline in LH, oestradiol and FSH. Ovulation then occurs. Ovulation is followed by a detectable rise in progesterone and oestradiol. Progesterone rises until day 20 (hence the rationale behind day 21 serum progesterones to test for ovulation in the average 28-day cycle with ovulation on day 14), plateaus until day 25 then falls to a low steady state by the start of menstruation. Oestradiol rises in the luteal phase until day 23 and then falls until menstruation. The luteal-phase endometrium forms lipid- and glycogen-rich subnuclear vacuoles 48 hours after ovulation. At 96 hours the vacuoles are supranuclear or luminal and release their secretions on day 20, which gives them a serrated appearance. There is a concomitant thickening of the endometrium due to an increase in glandular volume and stromal oedema, maximal on day 21. Predecidualization on day 23 consists of cytoplasmic enlargement of stromal cells around spiral arterioles and is accompanied by an increase in granulocyte and lymphocyte stromal infiltration.

Endometrial vasculature

The uterine arteries running up the lateral borders of the uterus give off branches which penetrate the lateral uterine walls, pass through the outer third of the myometrium and ramify into a ring of vessels known as arcuate arteries at the junction of the middle and outer thirds of the myometrium. Immediately prior to crossing the myometrial–endometrial border, they divide into basal and spiral arterioles. The basal arterioles supply only the basal endometrium and appear uninfluenced by the changes of the menstrual cycle, whereas the spiral arterioles are markedly influenced by the changes. They supply the superficial capillary bed of the endometrium and are therefore end arterioles. The uterine veins begin in the endometrium and run parallel to the glands, often with intercommunicating channels. They enter the myometrium, converge to form larger veins, and these in turn drain into arcuate veins, run parallel to the arcuate arteries and terminate in the uterine veins beside the uterine arteries. Menstrual blood loss is 50% arteriolar, 25% venous and 25% capillary and losses from diapedesis.

Further reading

Rees CMP, Barlow DH. Ovulation and the endometrial cycle. In: Turnbull Sir AC, Chamberlain GC, eds. *Obstetrics*. Edinburgh: Churchill Livingstone, 1989; 25–47.

Related topics of interest

Menarche (p. 70)
Menopause (p. 72)

MINIMALLY INVASIVE SURGERY

Advocates of minimally invasive surgery argue that patients benefit from a much shorter stay in hospital by comparison with those treated more conventionally. Opponents state that the same operation can be performed more safely and quickly by open means with only marginal increase in hospital stay. This topic will discuss hysteroscopic and laparoscopic surgery.

Hysteroscopy

The first attempt to visualize the inside of the uterine cavity was by Pantaleoni in 1869, but it wasn't until recently with the improvements in fibreoptics and instrumentation that hysteroscopy has become widely used. Prior to performing hysteroscopic surgery it is essential to gain experience in diagnostic hysteroscopy.

Some simple procedures can be performed at the same time as diagnostic hysteroscopy (for irregular, heavy or post-menopausal bleeding), including directional biopsies, removal of endometrial polyps and retrieval of lost IUCDs. It is now the investigation of choice compared to D&C.

Advanced procedures include division of uterine septae (laparoscopy is needed initially to exclude bicornuate uteri, and may be useful to assess tubal patency), division of adhesions causing Asherman's syndrome, endometrial resection, myomectomy and the development of sterilization methods.

Complications of hysteroscopic surgery include uterine perforation with visceral damage, fluid overload, infection and haemorrhage. Late complications include treatment failure, haematometra, pregnancy, and the possibility of the late presentation of endometrial carcinoma.

Advantages include a short hospital stay, rapid recovery, reduced morbidity and early return to work with reduced cost implications.

Laparoscopy

Professor K. Semm at Kiel in Germany was one of the first proponents of laparoscopic surgery in the 1970s. The first report of operative laparoscopy was in 1933 by Fervers, a general surgeon. Gynaecologists adopted laparoscopic techniques to perform sterilizations and the first laparoscopic hysterectomy was performed by Reich in 1989.

Laparoscopic surgery is advantageous when compared to laparotomy in that it avoids large uncosmetic, painful incisions with reduced postoperative analgesic requirements and hospital stay. There is less intraoperative blood loss, adhesion formation, tissue trauma and infection.

With regard to laparoscopic hysterectomy, it should be noted that this operation does not replace vaginal hysterectomy or necessarily make a difficult vaginal hysterectomy easier. Its role may be to convert an abdominal procedure to a vaginal one, or to allow the safe removal of the ovaries at the same time.

Laparoscopy does have complications with mortality rates of 3.7/100 000. Damage to vessels and viscera, CO_2 embolism and anaesthetic complications are known. The blind insertion of the Veress needle and trocar are responsible for the majority of vessel and visceral damage. Open laparoscopy (Hasson, 1971) involves a short incision through the skin, fascia and peritoneum prior to the introduction of the trocar under direct vision. About 4% of cases were done this way in the USA in 1982, despite the significant difference in terms of vascular and visceral damage.

The following are procedures that can be undertaken laparoscopically:

1. *Uterus*

- Repair of uterine perforation with or without removal of IUCD.
- Hysterectomy: total, subtotal, bilateral salpingo-uophorectomy (BSO), laparoscopically assisted vaginal hysterectomy (LAVH).
- Myomectomy.

2. *Adnexae*

- Adhesiolysis.
- Ectopic: salping-ostomy, -otomy, -ectomy.
- Ovarian cyst enucleation.
- Tubal surgery: reversal sterilization.
- Ovarian cystectomy, oophorectomy.
- Ovarian drilling: PCOD.

3. Endometriosis

- Endocoagulation.
- Division uterosacral ligaments.
- Laparoscopic uterosacral nerve ablation (luna).

4. Infertility

- IVF/GIFT/ZIFT.

5. Intra-abdominal

- Adhesiolysis.

6. Cancer

- Laparoscopic lymphadenectomy.
- Radical hysterectomy.

Further assessment of minimally invasive surgery is required to establish its final niche.

Further reading

DeCherney AH, Diamond MP *et al.* Endometrial ablation for intractable uterine bleeding: Hysteroscopic resection. *Obstetrics and Gynaecology,* 1987; **70:** 668–70.

Ewen SP, Sutton CJG. Laparoscopic hysterectomy: In: Studd J, ed. *Progress in Obstetrics and Gynaecology*, Vol 11. Edinburgh: Churchill Livingstone,1994; 261–71.

Goldrath MH, Fuller TA, Segal S. Laser photovapourisation of the endometrium for the treatment of menorrhagia. *American Journal of Obstetrics and Gynaecology,* 1981; **140:** 14–19.

Richardson RE, Magos AL. Laparoscopic hysterectomy: In: Studd J, ed. *Progress in Obstetrics and Gynaecology*, Vol 12. Edinburgh: Churchill Livingstone,1996; 355–78.

Semm K. Surgical pelviscopy: review of 12 060 pelviscopies, 1970–85. In: Studd J, ed. *Progress in Obstetrics and Gynaecology*, Vol 6. Edinburgh: Churchill Livingstone,

Related topics of interest

OVARIAN TUMOURS: EPITHELIAL

The vast majority of ovarian cancers, over 90%, arise from the epithelium. Benign tumours may present as enormous abdominopelvic masses causing the patient to appear cachexic, consistent with an advanced malignant state.

Ovarian cancer affects over 4000 women annually in England and Wales. It is estimated that over 75% of these women will die from the disease. The peak age of incidence is in the sixth and seventh decades and is related to the number of times a woman ovulates during her lifetime. Pregnancy, the oral contraceptive pill, late menarche and early menopause exert a protective effect.

Ovarian cancer is commoner in Western societies and there is a familial tendency for developing ovarian cancer. Predisposing genetic mutations are being identified, including the BRCA-1 gene (also increases the risk of breast cancer).

Pathology

Epithelial tumours may be benign or malignant and may resemble epithelia of structures which share a common developmental origin.

Serous tumours, resembling Fallopian tube epithelium, are the commonest, with the malignant variety accounting for 40–50% of epithelial cancers.

Endometrioid tumours are the second most common, accounting for 16–31% of cancers; this tumour may occasionally arise in a pre-existing focus of ovarian endometriosis, estimated to occur in 10–15% of cases.

Mucinous tumours, similar to endocervical glandular epithelium, in the malignant form account for 5–15% of epithelial cancers.

Other rare types are the clear cell tumours of Müllerian origin and the Brenner tumours, resembling uroepithelium, arising in cells of Wolffian origin.

A pathological concept unique to epithelial ovarian tumours is that of borderline malignancy in which there are histological features of malignancy but no frank invasion.

Diagnosis

Presentation is commonly at an advanced stage as early symptoms are non-specific. Late symptoms relate to the presence of a mass or ascites. Rarely a pleural effusion may be the presenting feature.

Treatment

The principle of treatment is to reduce tumour volume (cytoreductive surgery), aiming to leave no mass greater than 1 cm in diameter. This maximizes the efficacy of subsequent cytotoxic chemotherapy (carboplatin by a single IV infusion repeated 4-weekly for six courses, the dose being calculated by Calvert's formula).

Spread of disease is direct and by transperitoneal seeding, and optimal debulking may necessitate extensive intra-abdominal surgery with bowel resection a frequent requirement.

Standard treatment is total abdominal hysterectomy, bilateral salpingo-oophorectomy, omentectomy and appendicectomy. Other staging procedures, peritoneal washings for cytological analysis, para-aortic lymph node biopsies and random peritoneal biopsies may be indicated and lead to 'down-staging' of the disease.

Recurrent disease is rarely amenable to surgery. Second line chemotherapy is given; the choice of agent is dependent on the time from original treatment. A repeat course of carboplatin is more effective with a longer interval. Paclitaxel is a recently introduced agent shown to prolong survival in recurrent disease. Its use as first line therapy in combination with platinum is currently under investigation.

Screening

Methods available include; pelvic examination, ultrasound scan (abdominal, vaginal or colour Doppler), serum tumour marker (CA 125) and laparoscopy. The efficacy of large-scale population screening has not been proved. Screening for familial ovarian cancer is currently the subject of a national trial.

Fertility

The young woman with early-stage unilateral disease presents a difficult management dilemma. Conservation of the contralateral ovary and uterus, with definitive treatment delayed until child-bearing is complete, may be permitted if careful screening is employed and a thorough staging performed at the primary operation.

Borderline tumours generally present with stage 1 disease (usually unilateral) and may be managed in the same manner (if there is evidence of metastases then management is the same as frankly invasive cancer; prognosis is good).

Menopause

HRT may be given for menopausal symptoms after surgery for ovarian cancer. Endometrioid tumours are said to be oestrogen dependent. HRT is probably safe in this context, but patients should receive appropriate counselling.

Pseudomyxoma peritonei Benign mucinous tumours of intestinal type occasionally rupture with the release of mucin, which proliferates within the abdominal cavity, forming dense adhesions and a gelatinous mass that inhibit bowel motility and lead to intestinal obstruction.

Treatment is by laparotomy with debulking of any discrete tumour mass and evacuation of mucin, which is repeated as necessary.

Further reading

Calvert AH *et al.* Carboplatin dosage: Prospective evaluation of a simple formula based on renal function. *Journal of Clinical Oncology,* 1989; **7:** 1748–56.

Fox, H. Pathology of ovarian cancer. In: Shepherd JH, Monaghan JM, eds. *Clinical Gynaecological Oncology*, 2nd edn. Oxford: Blackwell Scientific Publications, 1990: 188–217.

Shepherd JH. Surgical management of ovarian cancer. In: Shepherd JH, Monaghan JM, eds. *Clinical Gynaecological Oncology*, 2nd edn. Oxford: Blackwell Scientific Publications, 1990: 218–46.

Related topics of interest

OVARIAN TUMOURS: NON-EPITHELIAL

Tumours of the germ cells and their supporting cells in the ovary give rise to a wide variety of tumours, particularly the former, which have the potential to differentiate along any cell line.

Management depends on accurate histological diagnosis. In general, these tumours tend to affect younger women, are diagnosed at an earlier stage and respond well to cytotoxic chemotherapy when compared with malignant epithelial tumours.

Secondary tumours of the ovary are relatively common because of the organ's well-developed blood supply and lymphatic drainage.

Germ cell tumours

These are commonly benign tumours (dermoid cysts) that occur in young women and exhibit a variety of cell types within the tumour, with formation of sebum a frequent feature. Occasionally they differentiate along solitary cell lines (monophyletic), e.g. a struma ovarii comprising functional thyroid tissue.

Malignant teratomata are related to the degree of immaturity of the constituent tissues, particularly mesenchyme and neuroepithelium. They metastasize readily and are markedly chemosensitive.

Malignant differentiation of primordial germ cells leads to dysgerminoma formation. Commoner in the 10–30 year age group, they readily metastasize in the abdominal cavity and via lymphatics. They respond extremely well to cytotoxic chemotherapy, and 90% of patients survive 5 years.

Differentiation to trophoblastic tissue gives rise to choriocarcinoma. Although rare, the outlook is poor as they do not respond to conventional treatment of uterine gestational choriocarcinoma.

Extraembryonic differentiation causes the rare yolk sac tumours. A tumour of young girls (4–20 years), they form large haemorrhagic masses which usually produce alphafetoprotein. Survival rates are much improved with cytotoxic chemotherapy.

Chemotherapy of germ cell tumours is with cisplatin, vinblastine and bleomycin. This highly toxic regimen has markedly improved survival figures in this group. Dysgerminoma responds well to the less toxic vincristine, actinomycin D and cyclophosphamide regimen, which has replaced radiotherapy as the treatment of choice.

Sex cord stromal tumours

Granulosa cell tumours are made up of granulosa and theca cells. The adult form is characterized by mainly solid tumours of low grade malignancy which may metastasize many years after primary treatment. They produce oestrogen and 5-year survival is of the order of 80%.

Juvenile granulosa cell tumour is a histological variant, about 5% of which behave in an aggressively malignant fashion.

Androblastomata are derived from primitive sex cord precursor cells which differentiate into Sertoli and Leydig cells. They are rare, usually small tumours, commonly benign, and produce testosterone.

Gynandroblastoma – this tumour is extremely rare and contains both Sertoli–Leydig and granulosa-thecal components mingled together.

The role of chemotherapy is uncertain, with poor response rates seen in aggressive malignancies.

Other stromal tumours

Fibromata are the commonest and may be included in the sex cord group. Usually solid tumours which are benign, they are the most likely tumours to be associated with a right hydrothorax in Meig's syndrome.

Other rare tumours include lipomata, haemangiomata and leiomyomata.

Secondary tumours

These mainly metastasize from the breast, colon and stomach, and both Krukenberg and non-Krukenberg tumours may arise from these primary sites.

Krukenberg tumours are a distinct histological entity, being mucinous adenocarcinomata with signet rings in a densely cellular stroma.

The prognosis for patients with metastatic ovarian cancer is extremely poor, with death within 12 months of diagnosis in the majority of cases.

Further reading

Fox H. Pathology of ovarian cancer. In: Shepherd JH, Monaghan JM, eds. *Clinical Gynaecological Oncology*, 2nd edn. Oxford: Blackwell Scientific Publications, 1990: 188–217.

Wiltshaw E. Chemotherapy of ovarian cancer. In: Shepherd JH, Monaghan JM, eds. *Clinical Gynaecological Oncology*, 2nd edn. Oxford: Blackwell Scientific Publications, 1990: 254–78.

Related topics of interest

Embryology (p. 205)
Gestational trophoblastic disease (p. 44)
Ovarian tumours: epithelial (p. 87)
Paediatric gynaecology (p. 93)

PAEDIATRIC GYNAECOLOGY

The neonate and infant

A mucous discharge, sometimes bloody, may come from the oedematous introitus as a result of increased cervical discharge and vaginal transudate caused by the transfer of maternal oestrogen to the fetus. 'Nappy rash', irritation and redness of vulva and buttocks generally infected by the bowel content, is an ammoniacal dermatitis caused by hot, wet nappies. Frequent nappy changes, regular skin washing and drying in warm air will help the majority. Sensitive skins will be helped by dimethicone cream 10%, gently massaged into the skin five times a day for a week and thereafter twice a day to waterproof the skin.

The young girl

Until the oestrogen surge a year before menarche the vagina is thin with no glycogen and no lactobacilli. It has a pH of 7.2. The oestrogen lack means that the vestibule and clitoral area are prominent; the vaginal orifice is barely seen or felt and hence infection is not usually a problem.

Infection

1. Vulvitis leading to secondary vaginitis. This is the most common form of infection associated with poor hygiene. Regular bathing, thorough drying and the use of loose cotton underwear will generally treat it.

2. Vaginitis leading to secondary vulvitis. This is uncommon and difficult to investigate. It may be the result of a congenital anomaly causing a vaginal discharge, e.g. ectopic ureter. The child may complain of burning on micturition, soreness or discharge; the mother may notice stained underwear.

3. General infection. This is usually from the bowel. *Gardnerella vaginalis* is the main microbe. Treat with local instillation of lactic acid 5%, with an eye dropper so as not to interfere with the hymenal ring. Other specific infections include:

4. Gonorrhoea. Below the age of 12 this is rare and implies sexual contact of some kind. If found it warrants admission. Search for other STDs. The contacts are usually family members. Treat with benzylpenicillin and probenecid.

5. Chlamydia. This is more common than gonorrhoea and the same rules apply. Do not treat with tetracyclines because of the dental effects.

6. Threadworms (Enterobius vermicularis). The worm is common, often carrying coliforms with it. Diagnose by the 'Sellotape' method or vaginal smear microscopy. Treat with mebendazole in those over 2 years of age.

7. Candidiasis. This is uncommon in young children and if found a medical reason should be sought, e.g. diabetes or antibiotics. Treat the very young with gentian violet 0.5–1.0% applied with an eye dropper. Nystatin suspension into the vagina with an antifungal on the perineum can be used in the older child.

8. Trichomoniasis. This is also uncommon and usually results from sexual contact. Treat with metronidazole.

9. Amoebiasis is common and is treated with metronidazole.

10. Viruses. Condyloma accuminata and herpes simplex can be seen. Condylomata are best treated with cryocautery, as podophyllin causes skin ulceration. Herpes simplex is rare in infants (apart from those whose mothers are excretors), and if found it implies sexual contact.

Foreign body

This is a common source of non-specific infection, vaginal discharge and/or bleeding. Rectal examination may detect the object and may facilitate 'milking' the object down to the introitus where it can be removed with a pair of nasal forceps. An EUA may be necessary. Sand from the beach picked up by naked children playing can be irritating and lead to infection. Gentle syringing with saline or lactic acid will treat it.

Ulcer

A round ulcer with a granular base, from which no organism can be cultured, and which when biopsied shows only granulation tissue, is known as a Lipschütz ulcer. It may occur at any age. Good hygiene is the best treatment and they usually disappear spontaneously.

Other forms of ulcerating vulval conditions, such as Behçet's syndrome, Crohn's disease and herpes are quite uncommon and require the appropriate immunological, histological and virological investigations.

Labial adhesions

These are relatively common, non-infective in origin and best treated with gentle outward pressure with the thumbs on the labia, followed by a little Vaseline for a few days.

Urethral prolapse

This is seen in 4–6 year olds. The prominent urethra plus tight underclothing and poor hygiene will result in a red, friable, bleeding urethral meatus. Diagnosis is confirmed by passing a catheter. An EUA and excision is the best treatment.

Trauma, allergies, skin diseases

These are other causes of paediatric gynaecological problems.

Sarcoma

Sarcoma botryoides is a highly malignant lesion, most common in the very young, <2 years of age, but it can be seen in older children. In younger children it presents with bleeding in a polyp or haemorrhagic mass in the lower vagina, and in older children it is seen higher in the vagina or at the cervix. Advanced cases will also have a palpable mass per abdomen. Rhabdomyoblasts are present. Management will include an EUA and cystoscopy and rectal examination, with chemotherapy being the initial treatment of choice. Surgery, in the form of a Wertheim's hysterectomy with a total vaginectomy, is indicated if tumour regression is incomplete after chemotherapy. Radiotherapy is sometimes used. These regimens result in a better prognosis than historically reported.

Further reading

Douglas CP. Vulvovaginal infection in young and old. In: Hare MJ, ed. *Genital Tract Infection in Women*. Edinburgh: Churchill Livingstone, 1988; 287–92.

Related topics of interest

PELVIC INFLAMMATORY DISEASE

This disease process results from infection of the upper female genital tract, in either the acute or the chronic phase.

Incidence

The exact incidence is unknown owing to the difficulty in ascertaining an infective cause in many women with pelvic pain and the fact that many women complaining of pelvic pain are wrongly labelled as having pelvic inflammatory disease.

Predisposing factors

Post-partum and post-abortal infection has been superseded as the commonest cause of PID by sexually transmitted diseases as a consequence of, on the one hand, improvements in maternity services and the effects of the 1967 Abortion Act and, on the other hand, contemporary sexual behaviour.

Any pelvic operation may lead to PID, particularly if any predisposing factors are present.

An IUCD is associated with an increased risk of PID.

Pelvic tuberculosis, a rare cause of chronic PID, is more commonly found amongst immigrants from the Indian subcontinent.

Pathology

Infective organisms may be endogenous or exogenous. The former group are implicated after childbirth and surgery and include vaginal and bowel commensals.

Bacteria commonly cultured from infective discharge include:

- Gram-negative rods, e.g. *E. coli*.
- Gram-positive cocci, e.g. beta-haemolytic streptococci (particularly in post-partum infection).
- Anaerobes, e.g. *Bacteroides* species.
- Sexually transmitted organisms, *Chlamydia* and *Neisseria gonorrhoea*.

Actinomyces israelii is a gut commensal occasionally cultured in PID associated with appendicitis or an IUCD.

Vaginal commensals such as *Gardnerella vaginalis* and *Mycoplasma hominis* are commonly found in association with pathogenic organisms but their primary role in the pathogenesis of PID is unclear.

Diagnosis

This depends on isolation of the causative organism(s) in the laboratory, in association with the typical clinical features of the disease.

Bacteriological investigation of endocervical swabs, blood cultures (repeated as necessary) and laparoscopic peritoneal aspirates may reveal the infective agents and provide antibiotic sensitivities. The last investigation is useful in doubtful cases and those which do not respond promptly to treatment.

Clinical features

1. Acute PID

Symptoms:

- Severe lower abdominal pain, worse on movement.
- Offensive vaginal discharge.
- The patient will feel generally unwell and feverish.

Signs:

- Fever with tachycardia, possibly associated with hypotension in the presence of septic shock.
- The lower abdomen will be generally tender with guarding and rebound tenderness.
- Pelvic examination is excruciatingly tender on both sides and cervical excitation tenderness is marked.
- An inflammatory mass may be palpable if the degree of tenderness allows.

2. Chronic PID

Symptoms:

- General malaise and fatigue.
- Chronic lower abdominal pain; may be constant with exacerbations, typically during menstruation.
- Intermittent offensive vaginal discharge.
- Deep dyspareunia.

Signs:

- Generalized lower abdominal tenderness, particularly on deep palpation. Pelvic tenderness, particularly cervical excitation tenderness. The presence of a bulky tender uterus and/or a tender adnexal mass of tubo-ovarian origin.

Investigations:

- Full blood count (leucocytosis and anaemia, the latter in chronic PID).
- ESR >100 mm/h in acute PID.
- Bacteriology as above.
- Laparoscopy (to confirm suspected cases, obtain fluid for culture, assess complicated or unresolved infection, drain an inflammatory mass or to assess chronic PID prior to a definitive procedure. The presence of perihepatic adhesions suggests the Fitz-Hugh-Curtis syndrome, associated with chlamydial infection.

Treatment

Antibiotics should be promptly administered in acute PID and modified in light of laboratory recommendations.

Therapy should initially aim to cover common pathogens with a broad-spectrum antibiotic combination.

Chronic PID may occasionally respond to a prolonged course of antibiotics.

Severe cases may require initial resuscitation and high-dose intravenous antibiotics.

Surgery is required to drain an infective collection in the pelvis; this may be performed laparoscopically.

Pelvic clearance may be necessary for refractory cases of chronic PID.

Tubal damage and infertility results from PID and prompt effective treatment is required to minimize this complication.

Further reading

Bevan C, Ridgeway GL. Pelvic inflammatory disease. *British Journal of Obstetrics and Gynaecology*, 1992; **99:** 944–5.

Whitfield CR. Pelvic inflammatory disease. In: MacLean AB, ed. *Clinical Infection in Obstetrics and Gynaecology*. Oxford: Blackwell Scientific Publications, 1990: 224–36.

Related topics of interest

PERIOPERATIVE COMPLICATIONS IN OBSTETRICS AND GYNAECOLOGY

Complications range from minor to life-threatening. They add greatly to the anxiety of the patient and relatives. Thorough knowledge of possible complications aids prompt recognition and allows appropriate management. Full and frank discussion with both patients and relatives at all stages of management minimizes anxiety for all concerned.

Problems

1. *Circulation.* Post-operative bleeding may be easily recognized if the site is readily apparent. Concealed (intra-abdominal) bleeding may not be apparent until the patient becomes shocked. Management is by careful observation of vital signs in the immediate post-operative period with prompt resuscitation followed by definitive treatment to arrest the haemorrhage. Delay in returning the patient to the operating theatre may lead to compromise of the renal circulation, followed by impairment of cardiac and cerebral circulation.

Prolonged slow bleeding may give rise to anaemia and delayed recovery or pelvic haematoma formation with pain and possible infection.

Thrombosis and subsequent embolism is relatively rare and may be adequately prevented with low-dose subcutaneous heparin. Established thrombosis is a potentially life-threatening condition, and prompt treatment with intravenous heparin is indicated.

2. *Respiration.* Atelectasis is a common event after general anaesthesia. It is usually accompanied by a transient pyrexia in the first 24 hours. Collapse of a small segment of lung usually resolves without further complication. Infection may supervene if the patient has existing pulmonary problems, is a smoker or is elderly. Complications are related to the duration of anaesthesia. The situation may be seriously exacerbated if pulmonary oedema occurs as a result of fluid overload, particularly in the high-risk groups. Careful monitoring of fluid balance is mandatory, particularly when intravenous fluids are administered for prolonged periods. Fluid balance is particularly important in the post-operative period in patients with pre-eclampsia in whom dramatic shifts between fluid compartments may occur.

Adult respiratory distress syndrome (ARDS) is a rare complication, related to prolonged and repeated anaesthesia and large-volume blood transfusion. Intensive supporting therapy is required, including positive pressure ventilation.

3. Cardiac. Myocardial infarction and cardiac failiure are the major complications, predisposed to by existing cardiac disease and fluid overload.

4. Infection. Any procedure may result in infection. This complication is minimized by careful aseptic and surgical technique. Prophylactic antibiotics are given in high-risk situations. Local infection is treated by exposure and irrigation. Treatment with antibiotics should commence when results of bacteriological investigations are available, unless the clinical situation warrants 'blind' treatment.

5. Trauma. Surgical trauma must be promptly recognized and repaired. Supportive measures such as prolonged catheterization and drainage for urinary tract injuries and defunctioning colostomy and drainage for bowel injuries must be employed where indicated.

Unrecognized urinary tract trauma leads to fistula formation. Conservative management with prolonged drainage of the urinary tract may effect a cure. Large fistulae or those refractory to conservative management require surgical correction.

Laparoscopic injuries require thorough assessment, preferably by laparotomy. Perforation of the uterus may be managed conservatively with regular observations.

Obstetric injuries require careful assessment and repair; adequate anaesthesia is necessary.

Timing of complications

1. Immediate. Trauma and haemorrhage may occur at operation; early recognition and prompt effective treatment are required.

2. Early. Haemorrhage, cardiac and respiratory complications occur in the first 48 hours after surgery. Careful attention to fluid balance, vital signs, urine output and analgesic requirements are necessary to minimize adverse effects. Predisposing problems such as diabetes mellitus must be adequately controlled.

3. Intermediate. In the first post-operative week thrombosis and infection may arise.

Paralytic ileus may become apparent at around the third day.

Wound dehiscence is more likely with a longitudinal incision; it may occur at any time in the first post-operative week. Predisposing factors include adverse factors which inhibit the healing process, e.g. hypoproteinaemia and poor surgical technique employed in wound closure.

A pelvic haematoma may present at or after the third day; spontaneous discharge is likely but abscess formation is a risk.

Further bleeding at 10–14 days is termed secondary haemorrhage and is particularly common after operations on the cervix, especially when infection supervenes.

Urinary tract fistula may present at any time in the first 2 weeks, commonly between the third day and the end of the first week. Intraperitoneal urinary leakage is a serious complication leading to severe pain and dense adhesion formation.

4. Late. Adhesions may cause pain and intestinal obstruction. Peritubal adhesions predispose to infertility.

Incisional hernia is commoner with midline incisions, particularly after severe wound infection.

Vault granulations occur after hysterectomy.

Prolapse and urinary incontinence may recur after corrective surgery.

Lymphatic collections occur after surgery to excise lymph nodes; these may be localized or diffuse, such as the lower limb after groin node dissection.

Uterine scars after Caesarean section may dehisce in a subsequent labour, particularly after classical section.

Further reading

Monaghan JM, ed. *Rob and Smith's Operative Surgery, Gynaecology*, 4th edn. London: Butterworths, 1983.

Related topics of interest

Abdominal versus vaginal hysterectomy (p. 1)
Caesarean section (p. 179)
Cancer of the cervix (p. 16)
Fistulae in obstetrics and gynaecology (p. 38)
Minimally invasive surgery (p. 84)
Pelvic inflammatory disease (p. 96)
Vulva (p. 151)

POLYCYSTIC OVARIAN DISEASE (PCOD)

In 1935, Stein and Leventhal described the syndrome of amenorrhoea, obesity and hirsuitism in seven women, with enlarged cystic ovaries. Polycystic ovarian disease (PCOD) is now known to be the commonest endocrine disorder in women of reproductive age. However, the symptoms are not specific and confusion may occur. In fact, 22% of the normal population may show polycystic ovaries. The prevalence amongst infertile women is approximately 5%, and it is the commonest cause of anovulatory infertility.

Aetiology

It is thought that abnormal gonadotrophin secretion (overproduction of LH relative to FSH) may induce hyperactivity of ovarian stroma, antral follicular atresia and disordered ovarian steroidogenesis, which in turn accentuates the LH hypersecretion.

Associations

PCOD is associated with hyperinsulinaemia in >75%. This confers a significantly increased risk of type II diabetes mellitus (non-insulin, late onset). Hypertriglycerideaemia, hypercholesterolaemia and hypertension with associated risk of premature cardiovascular disease are found in women with PCOD. Whether hyperinsulinaemia is cause or effect is unclear.

There are also well documented associations with the development of endometrial cancer, and also the occurrence of recurrent miscarriages.

Diagnosis

The diagnosis of PCOD may be made in a patient with the symptoms and signs of infertility, irregular periods, hirsuitism, obesity, DUB and virilization.

The investigations are based on determining the amount of androgenic hormones present. A simplified scheme for investigation is shown.

1. FSH/LH. Blood test taken within first 5 days of cycle. In PCOD reversed LH:FSH ratio of approximately 3:1

2. Testosterone. Raised in PCOD.

3. Oesterone. Raised in PCOD (>300 pmol/l).

4. Androstenedione. Raised in PCOD (>9.8 nmol/l).

5. Prolactin. Commonly found raised in 15% of patients.

6. Insulin I. Classically raised.

7. Ultrasound scan. The classic picture is of a necklace of small follicles all <5 mm in diameter positioned along the periphery of the ovary. The ovaries may be enlarged, or exhibit an increased amount or density of stroma.

8. Laparoscopy. Classically enlarged ovaries with a thickened white cover.

Differential diagnosis

- Acromegaly.
- Hyperthyroidism.
- Congenital adrenal hyperplasia.
- Cushing's syndrome.
- Hyperprolactinaemia.
- Anorexia nervosa and perimenarchal girls (USS appearance may be similar to PCOD).

Management

1. Hirsutism. This results from stimulation of the hair follicles by the excess androgens. Treatment is aimed at reducing this level.

(a) Cyproterone acetate is an anti-androgenic progestogen and combined with ethinyloestradiol is used for 6 months to suppress androgens. It is given in a dose of 2 mg with 35 µg of ethinyloestradiol. It is taken in the same way as the combined pill.

(b) GnRH analogues normalize the androgen levels after 1 or 2 months of treatment. They are as effective as cyproterone acetate in reducing hirsutism, but if add-back therapy utilizing a combined HRT with medroxyprogesterone acetate is used, reductions in hair growth of up to 50% can be achieved. GnRH analogues can also be successfully used when combined with the oral contraceptive pill, being more efficacious than the pill alone in improving gonadotrophins secretion and ovulation 6 months after stopping treatment.

Other treatment modalities such as the antiandrogen flutamide, spironolactone, dexamethasone, combined oral contraceptive pill and bromocriptine have been used, but in most cases women still remain hirsute. It is therefore important to include cosmetic remedies in this area of management.

2. Anovulation. Is the usual reason for infertility in women with PCOD. The first line of treatment is to use clomiphene citrate. Although often successful this may be associated with multiple follicular development, with an increase in the risk of multiple pregnancies. Some women are resistant to clomiphene and require gonadotrophin stimulation to induce ovulation. hMG (containing FSH and LH, ratio 1:1) or pure FSH (ratio FSH:LH 75:1) are used. GnRH agonists may be useful to normalize LH and FSH levels prior to gonadotrophin therapy, which needs careful monitoring [risks of ovarian hyperstimulation syndrome (OHSS)].

Surgical treatment has been advocated using bilateral wedge resection of the ovaries. Approximately a third of each ovary is removed and the ovary then reconstituted with meticulous haemostasis. 80–90% of women get regular menses, but conception rates are 45–60% and it may be associated with peritubal and ovarian adhesions. More recently the use of laparoscopic ovarian drilling has been advocated using diathermy or laser. Spontaneous ovulation has been reported in 92% with conception rates of 69%. Risks are damage to other organs, adhesion formation and ovarian atrophy.

3. Endometrial carcinoma. This is a potential complication for any woman in the presence of chronic oestrogen stimulation. Regular menses are therefore recommended and the use of the combined oral contraceptive pill or cyclical progestogens are used. It will protect the endometrium from becoming hyperplastic and will reduce hirsuitism; hence it often produces psychological benefit.

Further reading

Fox R. Polycystic ovarian disease and insulin resistance: Pathophysiology and wider health issues. In: Studd J, ed. *Progress in Obstetrics and Gynaecology*, Vol. 11. Edinburgh: Churchill Livingstone, 1994: 351–70.

Leventhal ML. The Stein-Leventhal syndrome. *American Journal of Obstetrics and Gynaecology,* 1958; **76:** 825–38.

McKenna TJ. Pathogenesis and treatment of polycystic ovary syndrome. *New England Journal of Medicine*, 1988; **318:** 558–62.

Murdoch AP. Polycystic ovary syndrome. *Hospital Update*, 1990; **16:** 643–4.

Related topics of interest

Hirsutism (p. 47)
Infertility – I (p. 57)
Infertility – II (p. 60)
Uterine tumours (p. 142)

PREMALIGNANT DISEASE OF THE CERVIX

Cancer of the cervix may be detected at a preinvasive stage by cytological examination of cells obtained from the transformation zone. An affected cervix can be examined by colposcopy and the abnormal area visualized after staining with dilute acetic acid and Lugol's iodine.

Invasive disease is excluded by histological examination of biopsy specimens, and the abnormal area is subsequently treated by excision biopsy (which may be combined with diagnostic biopsy) or local ablation.

Aetiology

A very strong association exists between invasive cancer and infection with human papillomavirus, strains, especially 16 and 18, also 31, 33 and 35. HPV is commonly found on the cervix in association with premalignant changes. HPV infection may regress spontaneously or cause progressive neoplastic change in cervical epithelial cells leading to invasive cancer.

Screening

Population screening by regular cervical cytology has been shown to reduce the incidence of invasive cancer. Introduction of a national computerized call and recall system in 1987 has increased the proportion of the target population screened and should lead to a reduced incidence in the near future in the UK.

Cytology

Accurate cytological reporting requires well-trained personnel.

Dyskaryosis is a term applied to cells in which changes in the size, colour and shape of cells, nuclei and cytoplasm suggest premalignant change.

Koilocytosis describes cells infected with HPV; they are enlarged, with irregular hyperchromatic nuclei and a perinuclear halo.

Smears in post-menopausal and pregnant women are often difficult to interpret. In the former a course of local oestrogen cream may allow satisfactory assessment.

Colposcopy

Adequate visualization of the entire transformation zone is the basis of a successful examination.

Application of acetic acid causes abnormal epithelium to appear white.

Punctation is seen when vessels proliferate and terminate in the abnormal epithelium; the coarser the punctuation the more severe the intraepithelial neoplasia. Similarly, these vessels may show a mosaic pattern of ramification in the abnormal epithelium.

Large irregular vessels in an area of raised epithelium suggest microinvasive disease.

Acetowhite change can occur with immature squamous metaplasia, the underlying columnar cells being outlined by the white change. Gland openings are seen in mature squamous metaplasia, which may also be outlined by acetowhite epithelium.

Areas of HPV infection exhibit acetowhite change, irregular areas, commonly with satellite lesions; they do not show the features of intraepithelial neoplasia.

Histology

Cervical intraepithelial neoplasia (CIN) is graded 1, 2 and 3, in increasing order of severity and, as such, is subject to observer variation in its diagnosis.

CIN may affect gland crypts, which on cut section may look like invasion.

Microinvasion is to a depth of 5 mm beneath the basement membrane; the lesion should not exceed 7 mm in its horizontal dimension. Larger lesions are termed frankly invasive.

Glandular lesions may occur, either in association with CIN or in a biopsy taken in response to abnormal glandular cells on smear. Glandular intraepithelial neoplasia may be graded as for CIN; the term adenocarcinoma *in situ* is also used.

Treatment

Local ablation may follow colposcopic-directed punch biopsies to exclude invasion. Alternatively, a larger biopsy sample is taken for both diagnostic and therapeutic purposes. A cone biopsy is indicated if the upper limit of the lesion cannot be visualized.

The former method has the disadvantage that the punch biopsy may not be representative and underlying invasive disease not adequately treated.

Excision biopsy can lead to a 'see and treat' policy, leading to more efficient management.

Local ablation may be performed with diathermy, cryocautery, 'cold' coagulation or laser vaporization. Complications include bleeding, superficial infection, irregular menstruation and rarely cervical stenosis.

Excision biopsy may be by LLETZ (large loop excision of the transformation zone) using a fine wire loop connected to an electrodiathermy unit. Adequate cone biopsies may be obtained under local anaesthesia using this method. This is the method of choice in the majority of units in the UK.

Cone biopsies may be taken using a carbon dioxide laser (more expensive, time-consuming, increased complications and an inferior quality of histological specimen compared with loop diathermy), or cut with a knife (general anaesthesia is required and the complication rate is higher, with cervical incompetence an added risk). Knife cone biopsies are infrequently performed, but may be indicated for persistently abnormal glandular cells.

Hysterectomy may be necessary if there is persistent dyskaryosis after local treatment or the cervix is unsuitable for local treatment (e.g. flush with the vaginal vault in a post-menopausal patient).

Further reading

Anderson MC. The pathology of CIN, VAIN and VIN. In: Shepherd JH, Monaghan JM, eds. *Clinical Gynaecological Oncology*, 2nd edn. Oxford: Blackwell Scientific Publications, 1990: 17–47.

Jordan JA. The management of CIN, VAIN and VIN. In: Shepherd JH, Monaghan JM, eds. *Clinical Gynaecological Oncology*, 2nd edn. Oxford: Blackwell Scientific Publications, 1990: 48–63.

Soutter WP. A practical approach to colposcopy. In: Studd J, ed. *Progress in Obstetrics and Gynaecology*, Vol. 7. Edinburgh: Churchill Livingstone, 1989: 355–67.

Related topics of interest

Cancer of the cervix (p. 16)
Sexually transmitted disease (p. 129)

PREMENSTRUAL SYNDROME

The premenstrual syndrome (PMS) consists of a group of behavioural, emotional and physical symptoms that recur during the second half of each menstrual cycle. These should abate completely after menstruation.

Only 5% of women will experience no premenstrual symptoms; however only between 20–40% will suffer symptoms severe enough to consult their doctor. Only 5% of such patients will be severely incapacitated with the symptoms.

Diagnosis

The diagnosis is dependent on timing the symptoms in relation to menstruation. Also, the presence of a symptom-free phase of at least 7 days after menstruation helps distinguish PMS from other menstrual problems. To help make a diagnosis, a women suspected of having PMS should keep a menstrual diary chart, giving daily ratings of common menstrual cycle symptoms.

A vast array of emotional and physical symptoms have been reported.

1. Emotional. Aggression, anxiety, depression, irritability, dysmenorrhoea, lack of concentration, crying bouts, change in libido, tension and fatigue.

2. Physical. Bloatedness, breast swelling and tenderness, headache, weight increase, swollen fingers and acne.

The cause of PMS is still unproven. However it would appear that hormonal events during the luteal phase play some part. Psychological factors are thought to be important although psychiatric disorders must be first ruled out. Other hypotheses are alterations in gonadal steroids, renin-angiotensin system, monoamine neurotransmitters and endogenous opioids, although none have been categorically proven.

Differential diagnosis

- Psychiatric disorders.
- Psychosexual problems.
- Causes of breast symptoms.
- Endometriosis.
- PID.

- Dysmenorrhoea.
- Lethargy/tiredness – anaemia/hypothyroidism.
- The menopause.

Treatment

Treatment is very difficult as the response to placebo is in excess of 90%, therefore everything else must be measured against this. For many women it is enough to have an understanding and sympathetic doctor who explains PMS to the woman.

Simple dietary advice has been used in the past such as maintaining a steady blood glucose, decreasing caffeine intake and salt intake.

Pyridoxine (Vitamin B_6) commonly used in doses of 50–300 mg/day. Thought to increase the levels of dopamine and serotonin. However long term use with doses over 25 mg/day has been associated with reversible peripheral neuropathy.

Oil of evening primrose contains linoleic acid, a polyunsaturated essential fatty acid, being the dietary precursor of several prostaglandins mainly E_2 and E_1. Their deficiency has been postulated to allow an enhanced response to β-endorphin, angiotensin II and ovarian hormones – hence administration may reverse this.

Progesterone and progestogens have been used on the basis that a deficiency of progesterone in the luteal phase caused PMS. However again no consistent evidence is available. Progestogens themselves may lower endogenous progesterone levels and cause symptoms similar to PMS.

Bromocriptine (up to 2.5 mg BD) has been used and is found to reduce cyclical breast pain and often other PMS symptoms, although again unsubstantiated.

Oestrogens are used in order to suppress ovulation on the basis that PMS is cyclical and that removal of the natural menstrual cycle will abolish PMS. This can be given as implants, the combined pill and oestrogen dermal patches; obviously regular courses of progesterones are essential to prevent endometrial hyperplasia. It has been found that this is one of the few methods of treatment that is better than placebo for all symptoms monitored.

Danazol has been used on a similar basis to oestrogen implants, in that it suppresses ovulation. The problem is that the doses required to suppress ovulation are associated with androgenic side effects and therefore with poor compliance.

Gonadotrophin-releasing hormone analogues (GnRH) have been used successfully in PMS, but continual usage cannot be recommended because of the unwanted effects of hot flushes, vaginal atrophy and osteoporosis. GnRH analogues with add-back HRT reduce the clinically relevant oestrogen responsive symptoms, but HRT is less efficacious in treating some of the other symptoms of PMS.

Other medications that have been used (and are still used) are *prostaglandin synthetase inhibitors* which were found to improve fatigue and discomfort; *prozac,* a selective serotonin re-uptake inhibitor, which has been shown to be extremely useful especially if the emotional symptoms predominate; *benzodiazepine* which was found to improve psychological symptoms only; *antidepressants* which only work when depression is the major symptom, and finally *diuretics* were advocated when symptoms of fluid retention were rife. However all these medications have no incontrovertible evidence to back up their use at present.

As a last resort it is theoretically possible to cure intractable symptoms by performing a hysterectomy along with a bilateral salpingo-oophorectomy. This will cure the PMS, but at some cost in terms of physical and psychological morbidity, mortality and continuous HRT.

Further reading

Managing the premenstrual syndrome. *Drug and Therapeutics Bulletin,* 1992; **30:** 69–72.

O'Brien PMS. Helping women with premenstrual syndrome. *British Medical Journal,* 1993, **307:** 1471–5.

Related topics of interest

PRURITUS VULVAE

Pruritus vulvae is marked and persistent itching of the vulva without any apparent primary cause. The itching does not involve the vagina and does not generally involve the anal area, whereas primary pruritus ani will tend to spread to the vulva.

Physiology

Itching sensory pathways are not well delineated. Pain and itch probably both arise in the free networks of nerve fibres without necessity for specialized end organs. Pain and itch are not synonymous, and itch is not subthreshold pain. The superficial plexus at the dermoepidermal junction is particularly involved in itching. It has been shown that the epidermis itself is not essential. The itch sensation is probably initiated by one or more chemical stimuli, produced either locally or elsewhere by vasodilatation or scratching damage. Prostaglandin E may be involved. Scratching will relieve 'normal' or 'physiological' itching as it causes large nerve fibre impulses to the central nervous system to override impulses from small nerve fibres. In pathological states similar stimuli result in earlier and more prolonged severe itching. Prolonged scratching liberates more irritants due to the trauma to the skin and hence a vicious circle is created.

Pathology

It is commoner in older women and is mostly seen after the age of 40 years. The main change seen is lichenification, and there may be secondary inflammation and infection. The most common causes are:

- Vulval dystrophy.
- Eczema due to an allergy.
- Vaginal discharge.
- Atrophic vaginitis.
- Threadworm.
- Diabetes.
- Uraemia.
- Liver failure.
- Pregnancy engorgement.
- Premenstrually.

Treatment

Where there is doubt about the diagnosis a vulval biopsy will be necessary. Remove any local source of allergy or irritation. Vulval soaps, douches and additions to the bathwater should be avoided, with simple soaps used to wash the skin and underwear. After washing gentle vulval drying with a hair dryer set on low may help. Loose-fitting cotton underwear without nylon tights is recommended. Steroids may be used, e.g. hydrocortisone 2.5% t.d.s. for a few weeks and thereafter hydrocortisone 1% should be sufficient. Night sedation may help break the cycle of nocturnal itch and scratch. Local anaesthetics and antihistamines will only further sensitize the area. HRT will relieve when atrophic causes are found. Any associated depression should be treated seriously and sympathetically.

Further reading

Soutter WP. Benign disease of the vulva and vagina. In: Shaw RW, Soutter WP, Stanton SL, eds. *Gynaecology*. Edinburgh: Churchill Livingstone, 1992; 385–95.

Related topics of interest

Bartholin's glands (p. 14)
Vaginal discharge (p. 145)
Vulva (p. 151)

RADIOLOGY

Ian Donald pioneered the introduction of ultrasound into obstetrics and gynaecology in the 1950s. The older technique of plain ionizing radiation to image the body has been largely superseded by the more recent advances in physics, electronics and computer technology.

Ultrasound

Ultrasound (US) waves are produced by applying a short electrical impulse to a piezoelectric crystal, causing it to change width, which in turn causes vibrations in the adjacent medium. The vibrations propagate through the medium as a pulsed, sinusoidal wave with amplitude, frequency and wavelength. The waves are reflected back to the transducer from the differing tissue interfaces and interpreted into recognizable structures on a video screen. In obstetrics and gynaecology the transducer may be used transabdominally, transvaginally or transrectally. There are various modes of US, including amplitude (A), brightness (B) (static and real time), and time-motion (TM). Three dimensional (3D) ultrasound is now widely available and is increasingly being used in clinical practice e.g. in reproductive medicine whilst imaging ovaries.

US may be used in obstetrics to assess the presence or absence of an intrauterine pregnancy, pregnancy gestation by GSV, CRL, BPD, HC, AC and femoral length, fetal morphology, placental site, maturity, morphology and degree of separation, AFV, umbilical cord site and structure, fetal and uteroplacental blood flow (often in conjunction with Doppler), fetal viability and presentation, number and zygosity of multiple pregnancy, site of entry for CVS or amniocentesis, cervical dilatation and fetal growth parameters. In gynaecology, US is useful in determining an adnexal mass with free peritoneal fluid and a thickened endometrium, i.e. an ectopic pregnancy, uterine fibroids, other tubal masses (e.g. hydrosalpinx), cervical, uterine and ovarian neoplasms (benign and malignant), the presence and site of an IUCD, retained products of conception after delivery and abortion or metastatic spread to the liver, diagnosis of hydatidiform mole and choriocarcinoma, associated structures such as the bladder, ureters, kidneys and liver. It has a special role in fertility management in assessing the site, size and number of ovarian follicles, egg retrieval and subsequent pregnancy progress in assisted conception. Contrast hysterosalpingography utilizing agents such as HyCoSy is in wide everyday clinical use to image Fallopian tube patency. Interventional ultrasound is increasingly being utilized to gain access to intraperitoneal structures such as ovarian cysts to either drain them or gain tissue for histopathological diagnosis.

US has not been found to be associated with any fetal damage at the macroscopic, microscopic or genetic level, nor has it been found to have any vertical transmission effects.

X-ray

Standard radiographs are produced by placing the patient between an X-ray source and photographic film. The resultant image is a shadow radiograph of the attenuation of X-ray photons by the patient. These films are crude images and often obscure structures vital to the diagnosis. Technological refinements are possible using radio-opaque contrast (e.g. IVU and angiograms) and computed tomography (CT).

X-ray, contrast enhancement and CT are used in obstetrics and gynaecology to assess pelvic morphology and dimensions (e.g. ELP), fetal bony morphology (e.g. dwarfing and osteogenesis syndromes), to locate an IUCD, and in hysterosalpingography and management of cervical, uterine and ovarian malignancy (tumour bulk, extragenital spread and node delineation – IVU, CT) and metastatic spread (liver and chest – CT and chest X-ray). Sophisticated variants of these techniques using specialized isotopes are used in radiotherapy to treat malignant tumours.

X-ray and its variants exposes patients to ionizing radiation that is potentially carcinogenic.

Magnetic resonance imaging

Magnetic resonance imaging (MRI) depends upon the magnetic properties of certain nuclei which, when placed within a magnetic field, and stimulated by radiowaves of a certain frequency, will absorb and then re-emit some of this energy as a radio signal. The modality is useful in delineating soft tissues in great detail, and the female pelvis is particularly suitable as it is little affected by respiratory motion. MRI can take sagittal or coronal views without moving the patient.

MRI in obstetrics and gynaecology is useful in ELP, and assessment of cervical, uterine and ovarian malignancies, including nodal and metastatic spread. It can also be used to follow the progress of a malignancy during radiotherapy and chemotherapy, or to diagnose recurrence at follow-up. It must be used with caution in epileptic patients and myocardial infarction patients (MRI is electroconvulsive and can cause atrial fibrillation) and it cannot be used in those with metal prostheses (e.g. patients with pacemakers and hip replacements). It is otherwise held to be safe, and poses no damage to the fetus after the first trimester.

Radionuclide imaging This provides more physiological detail than anatomical detail. It is used in bone imaging in oncology and ventilation-perfusion scanning in suspected pulmonary embolism. More recently radiolabelled monoclonal antibodies have been found useful in locating (radioimmunoscintigraphy) and treating (radioimmunotherapy) gynaecological cancers. It is a potentially carcinogenic modality.

Further reading

Chudleigh P, Pearce M. *Obstetric Ultrasound: How, Why and When.* Edinburgh: Churchill Livingstone, 1986.
Powell MC, Perkins A. Imaging techniques in gynaecology. In: Shaw RW, Soutter WP, Stanton SL, eds. *Gynaecology.* Edinburgh: Churchill Livingstone, 1992; 65–79.

Related topics of interest

Cancer of the cervix (p. 16)
Ectopic pregnancy (p. 28)
Ovarian tumours: epithelial (p. 87)
Ovarian tumours: non-epithelial (p. 90)
Uterine tumours (p. 142)

RADIOTHERAPY

Ionizing radiation causes injury to the genetic apparatus of a dividing cell, death of the cell occurring at subsequent mitosis. Cells with a high mitotic rate are preferentially killed.

The aim of radiotherapy is to deliver a lethal dose to the tumour while minimizing the damage to adjacent tissues.

Physics

The dose of ionizing radiation is that energy absorbed by a unit mass of tissue, the SI unit being the gray (Gy), which is equivalent to 1 joule per kilogram.

Ionizing radiation in gynaecological malignancy is delivered in two ways: via beam sources (external) and brachytherapy sources (internal).

Beam sources deliver radiation in the form of X-rays or gamma-rays. High-energy sources are preferred as they deliver the maximum dose at greater depth, which is essential for pelvic treatment. It is essential to know the dose delivered at a specific depth of tissue, and also the dose delivered to surrounding tissue, from a knowledge of the isodose curve at a given depth.

Brachytherapy sources are radionuclides placed in body cavities within or near to the treatment site. The commonly used source is caesium-137. The total dose required at each insertion is carefully calculated, and this determines the time the source is left *in situ*.

Radiobiology

Ionizing radiation affects genetic material but not the metabolic function of a cell.

Effects on tissues will depend on the rate of mitosis of the constituent cells.

Tumour cells have a rapid mitotic rate and consequently should be relatively radiosensitive. This is not true for all tumours for reasons which are incompletely understood. Hypoxic cells are relatively radioresistant, and the proportion of such cells in a given tumour will influence the response to treatment.

Normal cells show an early effect from radiation, with death in rapidly dividing cells such as intestinal epithelium and bone marrow. Later effects relate to a failure of the tissue owing to lack of replacement cells consequent upon depletion of the stem cell population. Supporting tissues are affected by fibrosis of connective tissue and ischaemia as a result of loss of endothelial cells.

Planning

Each patient is carefully assessed, with particular regard to the size and spread of the tumour, its relation to vital organs and the size of the patient.

The area to be irradiated may also include probable sites of metastatic spread, e.g. the pelvic side walls, where the pelvic lymph nodes are situated.

For external beam treatment the dose requirement and area to be treated are calculated from a series of X-rays taken with the patient on a simulator with identical movements to the external beam treatment machine.

Planning of brachytherapy treatment involves insertion of containers, moulds or needles with dummy sources, into the relevant site with the patient anaesthetized. The position and orientation of the sources may be checked by X-rays of the treatment site, followed by afterloading of the radioactive source, manually or via an afterloading machine.

Radiotherapy in gynaecology

Radiotherapy is utilized for primary treatment, adjuvant treatment, treatment of recurrent cancer and palliative therapy.

Radiotherapy is the primary form of treatment for patients with locally advanced cancer of the cervix. The results are generally similar to surgery in early-stage disease, but the latter treatment is generally preferred because of side-effects of irradiation.

Adjuvant radiotherapy is advised for pelvic nodal metastases or incomplete local excision of cervical cancer. Similarly, radiotherapy is given for regional nodal metastases in cancer of the vulva and corpus uteri as an adjunct to surgical excision.

Cancer of the vagina is commonly treated with radiotherapy, surgery being preferred for stage 1 and stage 4 disease.

Recurrent pelvic cancer, especially of cervix, may be amenable to radiotherapy, depending on the original treatment and the feasibility of exenterative surgery. Vaginal recurrence of an endometrial primary may be successfully treated by local insertion of irridium wires.

Palliative radiotherapy may be given to relieve pain or obstruction of blood and lymph vessels of the lower limb by tumour. It may also be given to relieve symptoms at distant sites.

Radiotherapy has been employed as an adjunct to surgery in carcinoma of the ovary, its use being largely superseded by platinum-based cytotoxic chemotherapy.

Further reading

Joslin CAF. Radiotherapy of the cervix, uterine corpus and ovary. In: Shepherd JH, Monaghan JM, eds. *Clinical Gynaecological Oncology*, 2nd edn. Oxford: Blackwell Scientific Publications, 1990; 371–412.
Pointon RCS, ed. *The Radiotherapy of Malignant Disease*, 2nd edn. London: Springer-Verlag, 1990.

Related topics of interest

Cancer of the cervix (p. 16)
Fistulae in obstetrics and gynaecology (p. 38)
Perioperative complications in obstetrics and gynaecology (p. 100)
Uterine tumours (p. 142)
Vaginal tumours (p. 148)
Vulva (p. 151)

REPORT ON THE NATIONAL CONFIDENTIAL ENQUIRY INTO PERIOPERATIVE DEATHS (NCEPOD)

Two reports by The National Confidential Enquiry into Perioperative Deaths, (NCEPOD), were released on the 30 September 1997. The 1994/95 Report of The National Confidential Enquiry into Perioperative Deaths covers perioperative deaths from the 1 April 1994 until the 31 March 1995. It covers 18 728 perioperative deaths, with a perioperative death being defined as a death under anaesthesia during surgery, or up to 30 days after surgery. The NCEPOD team scrutinized 1818 of these perioperative deaths, as a representative sample.

This report makes general recommendations relating to essential services (high dependency and intensive care beds), communication within and between specialties, specific circumstances (those >90 years of age, aortic stenosis, radical pelvic surgery, patients needing transfer to neurosurgical units, emergency vascular operations), improving organization of effective clinical audit, especially in gynaecology and ophthalmology, improving clinical records and data, and yet again assessing the abilities of locums.

In addition to the general recommendations, it makes many specific recommendations ranging from anaesthesia (e.g. SHOs working alone, problems in obtaining blood products), surgery (e.g. critical care services for paediatric surgery), pathology (e.g. Coronial referral rates, postmortem request rates), and to general data issues (e.g. loss of notes, return rate of NCEPOD questionnaires).

At the same time, the NCEPOD team released a second report, entitled 'Who Operates, When?' This report considered more than 50 000 surgical cases, with the principal aim being to assess emergency operating (especially out of hours), looking in detail at the time of surgery and the grade of anaesthetist and surgeon operating.

The recommendations and summary of findings make interesting reading, and should be added to previous reports and their findings.

The key points in the review of deaths with respect to anaesthetics were;
- Decision making was often unsatisfactory and made by too junior trainees.
- Perioperative management was sometimes poor, particularly in relation to preoperative resuscitation.
- Management of intravenous fluids was poor in some cases, with a lack of understanding of fundamental physiology appearing to be the problem.
- Records and charts were poorly kept or inadequate.

The key points in the review of deaths with respect to surgery were;

- There was a lack of preoperative preparation, particularly in relation to intravenous fluids, infrequent use of objective cardiac assessment, and patchy application of thromboembolic prophylaxis.

- There were a number of themes relating to suboptimal standards of delivery of care, particularly relating to delay in admission and surgery, too junior a surgeon operating, lack of communication between specialties, and inappropriate operations.

This report makes general and specific recommendations relating to admitting emergency surgical patients, the availability of year round, 24 hour operating rooms, other critical care services, appropriate staffing of such facilities, and the involvement of consultant staff. The recommendations will require implentation which in turn demands organizational changes (e.g. emergency operating lists, appropriately resourced, with rostered emergency anaesthetists and surgeons being free of other commitments, a designated theatre arbitratror to decide on case priority, an operating theatre record of all staff present with each case, systematic audit of theatre patterns of work, a harmonization of clinical definitions used by surgeons and anaesthetists), and clinical changes (optimizing patient conditions before submitting them to anaesthesia and surgery, local protocols relating to preoperative starvation, fluids, analgesia, the elderly and ICU and HDU facilities).

The reports together make mandatory reading for all engaged in anaesthesia and surgery, and regrettably repetitively make many points covered in previous reports.

Further reading

Campling, EA, Devlin, HB, Hoile, RW, Ingram, GS, Lunn, JN, eds. *Report of The National Confidential Enquiry into Perioperative Deaths, 1994/95.* London: National Confidential Enquiry into Perioperative Deaths.

Campling, EA, Devlin, HB, Hoile, RW, Ingram, GS, Lunn, JN, eds. *Who Operates, When? A Report by the National Confidential Enquiry into Perioperative Deaths, 1 April 1995 to 31 March, 1996.* London: National Confidential Enquiry into Perioperative Deaths.

Related topics of interest

Ectopic pregnancy (p. 28)
Report on Confidential Enquiries into Maternal Deaths in the United Kingdom, 1991–1993 (p. 309)

RISK MANAGEMENT

Risk management is the process of reducing or eliminating losses due to accident or misadventure. Such events are known as incidents; an incident may result in injury/adverse outcome to:

- a patient
- a member of staff
- a member of the public.

Individual doctors are advised to be aware of the principles of risk management, and in no field of medicine is this more important than obstetrics and gynaecology. There is a growing body of evidence that patients in the United Kingdom are beginning to adopt American style approaches to medical procedures, and in particular towards litigation when patient outcomes are less than satisfactory. The Clinical Negligence Scheme for Trusts (CNST), which is open to all health care Trusts in the United Kingdom, reported 634 'open' claims against Trusts in the summer of 1997, with an estimated value of £180 million. It is held that the true figure will be £500 million once incidents which are yet to be reported are taken into account. Obstetric claims make up by far the largest quantum, being estimated at £60 million in the summer report. The CNST is designed to optimize patient care and protect Trusts against the adverse consequences of clinical negligence. In so doing, Trusts have an obligation to adopt appropriate measures to ensure medical staff are clinically competent, but the principles of risk management are primarily incumbent upon individual doctors as they go about their daily work.

Doctors can reduce the danger of therapeutic mishaps or adverse outcomes, and hence reduce the possibility of legal proceedings if they adopt the five 'Cs' approach:

1. Communication
2. Counselling
3. Consent
4. Competence
5. Case notes.

In obstetrics and gynaecology there are a number of trigger events that should alert medical staff to initiate the risk management protocol of the Trust, which in itself is part of a wider concept known as quality assurance. Typical examples of such incidents are:

Trigger incidents in risk management schemes	
Obstetrics	Gynaecology

Neonatal encephalopathy
  in term babies
Undiagnosed fetal abnormalities
Stillbirth or neonatal death
Erb's palsy
Unexpected or late SCBU admission
Failed forceps/Ventouse
Delivery interval for Caesarean section
  of greater than 40 minutes
Serious maternal complications
Readmission to hospital
	Failed sterilization
	Failed termination
	Perforated uterus
	Anuria after
	  hysterectomy
	Peritonitis after
	  laparoscopy

In addition individual doctors will need to consider whether or not they should have independent medical insurance of the type offered by The Medical Defence Union and The Medical Protection Society.

Finally, when something does go wrong, a swift and sympathetic response, with an apology and an admission of regret (without a need to admit negligence in the first instance) are sometimes all that are needed to avoid a potentially damaging and costly legal dispute.

Further reading

Chamberlain, G. *How to Avoid Medico-Legal Problems in Obstetrics and Gynaecology*, 2nd edn. London: RCOG, 1992.

Clements, RV. *Safe Practice in Obstetrics and Gynaecology*. London: Churchill Livingstone, 1994.

Vincent, C. *Clinical Risk Management*. BMJ Publications, 1995.

Related topics of interest

SEXUAL FUNCTION

Normal sexual experience is dependent upon intact pelvic organs with functioning vascular and neurological mechanisms. All changes due to sexual arousal are irrevocably linked with cognitive processes.

Anatomy and physiology

Masters and Johnson's classification divides human sexual response into four phases:

- Excitement.
- Plateau.
- Orgasm.
- Resolution.

This classification does not take into account libido or desire, which is a vital part of any sexual dynamics. Each phase is incremental upon the preceding, and each is necessary for the subsequent phase to occur. Each phase has genital and systemic components, e.g. changes in colour and size of the labia and vagina and penis, increase in pulse, respiratory rate and blood pressure. The corticosensory experience of orgasm represents the peak of the pleasurable sensation of sexual activity, but is not necessary in either the male or female for fertilization to occur.

Female sexual dysfunction

- Dyspareunia/apareunia.
- Vaginismus.
- Orgasmic dysfunction.
- General sexual dysfunction.

Male sexual dysfunction

- Primary or secondary erectile difficulty.
- Premature ejaculation.
- Dyspareunia.
- Other ejaculatory dysfunction.

Aetiology

In up to 50% of cases erectile problems have an organic cause. It is thought that many female problems are psychological in origin, but the true percentages are unknown. Consider neurological conditions (e.g diabetes, multiple sclerosis, spinal cord injury), previous surgery, especially for gynaecological cancer, and the post-hysterectomy syndrome. Drugs may be implicated, especially alcohol. Dyspareunia and apareunia after childbirth are relatively common, and all gynaecologists are familiar with having to re-repair the perineum, vulva and vagina after an episiotomy which has healed incorrectly.

Epidemiology

Many never present with their problems. Kinsey found that at least 10% of women in their thirties are anorgasmic, with male sexual function deteriorating with age. Orgasmic dysfunction does not necessarily mean sexual dysfunction, and a normal physiological sexual experience does not preclude sexual dysfunction. It is believed that gynaecological clinic attendees have higher than average sexual dysfunction, with female attendees more likely to complain of loss of enjoyment, whereas male attendees complain of loss of genital function. In at least one-third of couples, in which one partner in a relationship complains of sexual dysfunction, the other partner will be found to also have a problem.

Diagnosis

This will follow a recognition that there is a problem. A frank and detailed sexual history and then a careful physical examination are required. Check for normal secondary sexual characteristics and possible causes, e.g. infection and poorly sutured episiotomy scars. Twenty per cent of women have a retroverted uterus which can be a cause of deep dyspareunia. Chronic pelvic infection and endometriosis may warrant treatment.

Treatment

In the absence of organic pathology, a structured approach is necessary. Education about anatomy and physiology may be necessary with some couples, and the perimenopausal and post-menopausal woman may need HRT or vaginal lubrication advice. Modern intensive sexual counselling is mostly behaviour based, e.g. sensate focus, which initially 'bans' sexual intercourse. Time, empathy, communciation and confidentiality are of the essence in the relationship between a couple and between the couple and the therapist.

Results

Assessment of 'success' is difficult. It is believed that 65% will report at least an improvement after intensive sexual counselling, but many studies have shown a high relapse rate.

Further reading

Parsons A. Psychosexual disorders. In: Shaw RW, Soutter WP, Stanton SL, eds. *Gynaecology*. Edinburgh: Churchill Livingstone, 1992; 843–50.

Related topics of interest

Hormone replacement therapy (p. 50)
Menstrual cycle physiology (p. 81)
Puerperal psychosis (p. 298)

SEXUALLY TRANSMITTED DISEASE

The term sexually transmitted disease applies to infection which is specifically transmitted by sexual contact.

Acquired immune deficiency syndrome and hepatitis B are commonly acquired by sexual contact, although at present in the United Kingdom the commonest route of transmission in women is sharing of infected needles by intravenous drug abusers.

Syphilis

The incidence of syphilis has been relatively low since the late 1980s, with 304 cases in England in 1994 (the majority in men). It is expected to rise in the near future, reflecting an increased incidence in Eastern Europe.

The causative organism is the spirochaete bacterium *Treponema pallidum*. Spirochaetes cause the related infections yaws and pinta.

Primary syphilis causes a local (usually genital) ulcer or chancre to appear, followed by a secondary or systemic stage characterized by a rash, malaise, mucosal (snail track) ulceration and condylomata lata.

Tertiary syphilis may affect the nervous or cardiovascular systems with progressive destructive lesions or gummata.

The spirochaete crosses the placenta and leads to congenital syphilis (one case in 1983) with widespread infection in a proportion of affected babies.

Diagnosis is by serological tests; the VDRL measures antibody to treponemal cardiolipin antigen and the TPHA to other treponemal antibodies. These are non-specific and definitive diagnosis is by fluorescent treponemal antibody testing, which is unsuitable for screening.

Treatment is with Bicillin (procaine penicillin and benzylpenicillin) given intramuscularly. Erythromycin is an alternative.

Gonorrhoea

Gonorrhoea is a worldwide problem; the incidence is rising in England and Wales with 3786 reported cases in women in 1996.

It is caused by the Gram-negative diplococcus *Neisseria gonorrhoea*. It is highly infective and affects the lower genital tract, urethra and rectum, causing an irritation and discharge. It commonly ascends in the pelvis to produce acute pelvic inflammatory disease, resulting in severe adhesions and possibly abscess formation and systemic spread. It may also cause a Bartholin's abscess, ophthalmia neonatorum and monoarticular arthritis.

Diagnosis is by culture of urethral, endocervical and rectal swabs, preferably charcoal swabs, transported in Stuart's enriched medium and incubated in a carbon dioxide-rich environment.

The majority of strains of the bacterium remain sensitive to penicillin, although beta-lactamase-positive strains which respond to cephalosporins or gentamicin are emerging. It is common for an associated chlamydial infection to occur, especially with pelvic sepsis, which should be treated concurrently.

Chlamydia

Chlamydia trachomatis is an obligate intracellular parasite containing both DNA and RNA, and therefore having characteristics of both bacteria and viruses. Urogenital infection is caused by the subtypes L1, L2 and L3.

Chlamydial infection may cause little in the way of symptoms: discharge from the vagina and cervix; mild pelvic discomfort or dysuria. The organism is often found in conjunction with gonococcal infection and causes perihepatic adhesions of the Fitz-Hugh-Curtis syndrome, by intraperitoneal spread from a pelvic focus of infection.

Chlamydia has been notoriously difficult to detect in the laboratory, but the development of an enzyme-linked immunosorbent assay has improved the diagnostic accuracy.

The drug of choice in chlamydial infection is doxycycline.

Genital herpes

The DNA virus herpes simplex has two main subtypes, 1 and 2, both of which may infect the genital tract, the majority of cases being due to HSV 2.

There were 26 800 reported cases in England in 1994 – a rising incidence.

A primary attack causes tingling and burning sensations in the infected area followed by the appearance of small vesicles on the cervix, vagina or surrounding skin. These may be associated with excruciating pain.

The primary infection slowly resolves, and the virus migrates via sensory nerves to the sacral ganglia, where it remains quiescent until reactivation occurs.

Stimuli to reactivation include systemic illness, immunosuppression, fatigue, stress and menstruation.

Recurrent attacks are generally milder, complications are rare and include meningitis, proctitis and whitlows.

Diagnosis is on clinical grounds, aided by microscopy and culture of infected vesicular fluid and swabs.

Treatment is with acyclovir or famciclovir, oral or parenteral. Treatment is more effective if commenced as soon as prodromal symptoms appear. Famciclovir is said to reduce the incidence of recurrent attacks.

Genital warts

Genital warts are caused by infection with a small DNA virus, HPV, of which there are many subtypes. Types 6 and 11 are commonly associated with genital warts.

Condylomata may be raised or flat, the latter associated with itching.

Warts may regress spontaneously or may enlarge significantly, commonly in pregnancy. There is an association with wart virus infection and the development of cervical and vulval cancer.

Diagnosis is on clinical grounds or by histological examination of biopsy material.

Treatment is by podophyllin applied to the affected area (contraindicated in pregnancy) or by local ablation with the laser or diathermy.

Further reading

McMillan A. Sexually transmitted diseases. In: Studd J, ed. *Progress in Obstetrics and Gynaecology*, Vol. 5. Edinburgh: Churchill Livingstone, 1985; 309–31.

Roberts J. Genitourinary medicine. In: MacLean AB, ed. *Clinical Infection in Obstetrics and Gynaecology*. Oxford: Blackwell Scientific Publications, 1990; 237–54.

Related topics of interest

THERAPEUTIC ABORTION AND THE HUMAN FERTILIZATION AND EMBRYOLOGY ACT 1990

In the United Kingdom, a spontaneous abortion is defined as a pregnancy loss occurring before 24 completed weeks of gestation. WHO defines an abortion as as the expulsion or extraction from its mother of a fetus or an embryo weighing 500 g or less. This latter definition therefore incorporates provision for therapeutic abortion by virtue of the words 'or extraction'.

Therapeutic abortion

Therapeutic termination of pregnancy (or induced abortion) is the term used to describe medical or surgical termination of pregnancy. There were 163 638 such terminations performed in England and Wales in 1995, a 2% decrease on the 1994 figure. They account for about 20% of all pregnancies per year. At least 85% are performed in the first trimester, the upper limit for 'social' termination being 24 weeks. Counselling, contraceptive advice and identification of high-risk patients (teenagers, repeat terminations, sexually abused patients, late terminations) are an integral part of the pretermination process.

Methods

1. *First trimester*
   (a) Medical using mifepristone (RU 486) and misoprostol before 9 weeks gestation. This regimen should result in at least a 90% complete abortion rate, with <5% requiring ERPOC.
   (b) Surgical using misoprostol and followed by uterine evacuation under anaesthesia.

2. *Second trimester*
   (a) Medical using mifepristone and misoprostol, or variants e.g. gemeprost, and IV syntocinon and/or extramniotic prostaglandin.
   (b) Surgical dilatation and evacuation up to 18 weeks is performed by some.
   (c) Hysterotomy is now rarely used.

Complications

1. *RPOC.* The frequency is up to 5%.

2. *Perforation.* Small perforations require no action other than observation, but rarely a large perforation can

involve the bowel. This will require a laparotomy and a colorectal surgeon. If in doubt laparoscopy should be performed.

3. Haemorrhage. Blood loss with a termination increases with gestation, being around 50 ml at 8 weeks and 100 ml at 12 weeks. Losses >500 ml are significant and will require careful assessment and possible re-evacuation, oxytocics and blood transfusion. Rarely hysterectomy may be necessary.

4. Infection is uncommon and is mostly due to RPOC. Antibiotics and possible re-evacuation will be required.

5. Cervical trauma can lead to either stenosis or incompetence.

6. Psychological damage is not uncommon in the form of guilt, loss, grief and depression. Pretermination counselling may identify those at risk.

7. Infertility is rare after termination. Infection may have led to tubal damage and this should be looked at early.

8. Rhesus isoimmunization may occur if anti-D is not given to Rhesus-negative women after termination.

The Human Fertilization and Embryology Act 1990

Therapeutic termination of pregnancy is governed by specific legislation incorporated in the The Abortion Act of 1967 and The Human Fertilization and Embryology Act (HFEA) of 1990. These two Acts supersede the Infant Life (Preservation) Act of 1929 with respect to termination of pregnancy. There are four clauses permitting such an abortion, ranging from risk to maternal well-being in physical and mental health terms, risk to the child if it were born, substantial risk of serious fetal anomaly and grave concern for the life of the mother. There are statutory legal requirements incumbent upon the two medical practitioners certifying each case, and the data are collected and analysed by the Department of Health. The legislation as it now stands enables a termination of pregnancy to be performed at any gestation, but only in an NHS hospital if the gestation is >24 weeks; private hospitals and clinics may perform terminations <24 weeks. Clause 38 specifically permits conscientious objection to any Act-related activities.

Other aspects of HFEA The main aim of HFEA is to make provision in connection with human embryos and any subsequent development of such embryos; to prohibit certain practices in connection with embryos and gametes; to establish a Human Fertilization and Embryology Authority (entrusted to ensure compliance with the Act and to license institutions involved with Act-related activities); to make provision about the persons who in certain circumstances are to be treated as the parents of a child; and to amend the Surrogacy Amendments Act 1985. The law in this area continues to be dynamic and evolving as evidenced by the recent High Court decisions relating to the use of sperm taken after brain death and the issue of consent; the Diane Blood case.

Further reading

Edmonds DK. Spontaneous and recurrent abortion. In: Shaw RW, Soutter WP, Stanton SL, eds. *Gynaecology*. Edinburgh: Churchill Livingstone, 1992; 205–18.
Newton J. Contraception, sterilisation and abortion. In: Shaw RW, Soutter WP, Stanton SL, eds. *Gynaecology*. Edinburgh: Churchill Livingstone, 1992; 291–312.
The Abortion Act 1967. HMSO: London.
The Human Fertilisation and Embryology Act 1990. HMSO: London.

Related topics of interest

URINARY INCONTINENCE: INCONTINENCE AND RETENTION

Urinary incontinence is defined as a condition with involuntary loss of urine causing a social or hygiene problem. Up to 50% of young healthy nulliparous women wet themselves occasionally.

Causes

- Genuine stress incontinence (GSI).
- Detrusor instability.
- Urethral instability.
- Overflow incontinence.
- Fistulae – malignant or iatrogenic.
- Congenital anomalies.
- Functional.
- Miscellaneous.

GSI

This is the commonest cause, accounting for 60% of cases, with symptoms of stress, urge, urgency and frequency. It is defined as involuntary loss of urine when the intravesical pressure exceeds the maximum urethral pressure, in the absence of detrusor activity. It can really only be diagnosed at urodynamics, as stress as a symptom or a sign is not pathognomonic of GSI. Conservative treatment with pelvic floor physiotherapy is useful when used in conjunction with perineometry and/or vaginal cones. Post-menopausal patients may benefit from oestrogen. Colposuspension is the operation that gives the best long-term results (85–90% continence in the right cases) but it may give the patient continence with frequency and urgency, i.e. detrusor instability symptoms. Many other operations are available ranging from vaginal approaches (e.g. anterior colporrhaphy) to peri- or transurethral approaches (e.g. collagen or vulcanized silicone implants) to combined abdomino-vaginal approaches (e.g. Stamey or Pereyra-Raz) to other abdominal approaches (e.g. urethral sling procedures using endogenous or exogenous materials). Each has their exponents, with the best results occurring in experienced surgeons' hands who have chosen wisely for the particular patient's circumstances. Such operations may be combined with other procedures being undertaken, e.g. colposuspension and abdominal hysterectomy or vulcanized silicone implants with vaginal hysterectomy.

Detrusor instability

Detrusor instability is the second most common cause of incontinence, with symptoms of stress, urge, urgency, enuresis, frequency and nocturia.The urethra functions normally, but the detrusor behaves in an uninhibited manner, causing intravesical pressure to exceed the urethral pressure. Also known as unstable, uninhibited, hyperreflexic or dyssynergia. The diagnosis may only be made at urodynamics with a detrusor pressure rise >15 cm H_2O at filling or provocation. The aetiology is often unclear, but it may be a presentation in neurological disease such as multiple sclerosis. Treatment is with anticholinergics and/or bladder training. It may coexist with GSI, in which case one should treat the detrusor problem first on the premise that a reduction in detrusor pressure will relieve the incontinence. If this fails, surgery may be considered, but the results are not as good as with pure GSI alone.

Urethral instability

This newly diagnosed entity has as yet no known treatment.

Overflow incontinence

This uncommon condition is due to urethral obstruction or detrusor inactivity, and is defined as an involuntary loss of urine when the intravesical pressure exceeds the maximum urethral pressure because of an elevation of intravesical pressure associated with bladder distension, but often in the absence of detrusor activity. It presents as continual dribbling or low voiding volumes in conjunction with stress. It is often diagnosed by the large palpable bladder, or at cystometry. The differential diagnosis includes drugs, upper motor neurone lesions, regional anaesthesia, surgery, a pelvic mass or genital inflammation, with the treatment tailored accordingly.

Fistulae

All forms of pelvic fistulae cause incontinence. It is always constant incontinence, regardless of time. In the western world it is usually iatrogenic following surgery and/or radiotherapy or due to malignancy, whereas in developing countries it is usually the result of obstructed labour and poor obstetrics.

Congenital anomalies	These are not always diagnosed at birth or in infancy. The treatment will depend upon the diagnosis, but will mostly be surgical.
Functional	One-third of such cases will respond to psychiatric intervention, but this should only be resorted to when organic pathology has been excluded.
Miscellaneous	These include minor anomalies such as a urethral diverticulum, or sensory urgency due to an atrophic epithelium in the post-menopausal age group. This latter group should respond to oestrogen therapy.
Voiding difficulties	Most commonly these are the result of poor detrusor activity, which can be rectified with cholomimetic agents such as bethanecol. Alternatively, intermittent self-catheterization is convenient and easily taught to the majority, and surprisingly has a low infection rate. Phenoxybenzamine may be useful for detrusor sphincter dyssynergia.
Urinary retention	This may occur for a number of reasons:

1. Outlet obstruction. Cervical or ovarian mass.

2. Detrusor inactivity. See overflow incontinence and voiding difficulties.

3. Pregnancy. Retroverted gravid uterus in the second trimester. In the third trimester an engaging fetal head may cause outlet obstruction with incomplete emptying.

4. Post-traumatic. Most commonly seen after an epidural anaesthetic, Caesarean section or operative vaginal delivery causing a temporary denervation of the bladder.

5. Post-operative. After abdominal or vaginal bladder repair surgery.

6. Neurological. Sacral spinal cord lesions, upper motor neurone lesions, syphylitic bladder, multiple sclerosis.

7. Drugs.

| **Treatment** | Initial treatment will always consist of bladder emptying with a catheter, and then tailored treatment depending upon the underlying cause. |

Further reading

Cardozo L. The use of cystometry in the understanding of urinary incontinence. In: Studd J, ed. *Progress in Obstetrics and Gynaecology*, Vol. 1. Edinburgh: Churchill Livingstone, 1981; 151–66.
Stanton SL. The abdominal approach for the treatment of urinary incontinence. In: *Studd J, ed.* Progress in Obstetrics and Gynaecology, Vol. 1. Edinburgh: Churchill Livingstone, 1981; 167–81.

Related topic of interest

Urinary incontinence: urodynamics (p. 139)

URINARY INCONTINENCE: URODYNAMICS

Urodynamics may be defined as the science of urinary flow, but in more general terms it has come to mean all the investigations used by urologists and gynaecologists to assess the function of the lower urinary tract. It may at times be extended to assess the upper urinary tract. The bladder's dual roles of storage and expulsion of urine lead to assessments of urinary continence and voiding dysfunction. Up to 50% of women may be affected with a continence or voiding problem at some time in life.

	Symptoms		
Tests	Incontinence	Urgency/frequency	Voiding difficulty
History, examination and MSU	+	+	+
Pad test	+		
Uroflowmetry	+		+
Videocystourethrography	+	+	+
Urethral pressure profile		+	+

Initial assessment

All urinary tract assessment must begin with a thorough history and examination to ascertain the nature, severity, anatomy and possible pathophysiology. Infection must be excluded and eradicated before proceeding to urodynamic investigation. A thorough drug history is essential as many drugs are linked to urinary problems, e.g. diuretics can lead to frequency, and equally concomitant conditions such as chronic obstructive airways disease, multiparity and obesity may predispose to cough-induced urinary incontinence.

All patients presenting for urodynamic evaluation should have completed a urinary diary, preferably over a week, recording time and volume of intake and output, and related symptoms and signs such as urgency or incontinence.

Methods available

1. Flow studies. The patient, with a comfortably full bladder, voids in private through a flowmeter. A rate of >15 ml/s is normal. A low flow rate needs to be reproduced on more than two occasions if any meaning is to be attached to it. Low flow rates may be due to outlet obstruction or poor detrusor contractility.

2. *Quantifying urinary loss.* This may be elicited by provocation in the laboratory, e.g. patient coughs or jumps up and down with a full bladder, but more accurately is done via nappy, pad, urethral urinary detection or 24 hour home pad tests.

3. *Cystometry.* The oldest and most useful test, cystometry measures the intravesical pressure during different urinary states. The detrusor pressure (DP) can be calculated thus:

$$P_{det} = P_{ves} - P_{abd},$$

where, P_{det} = Detrusor pressure
P_{ves} = Intravesical pressure
P_{abd} = Intra-abdominal pressure.

Intra-abdominal pressure is approximated from an intrarectal pressure transducer and intravesical pressure is measured by an intravesical pressure transducer located within a fine gauge catheter. Cystometry may be divided into the filling phase, which may elicit aberrant detrusor activity, and the voiding phase which may assess detrusor contractility. Normal women void with low detrusor pressure (i.e. <15 cm H_2O). The results of such studies may be graphically and dynamically plotted on a cystometrogram.

4. *Videocystourethrography.* This employs radiological screening during cystometric assessment, so that in addition to the normal cystometry parameters, the anatomy and function of the lower urinary tract may be seen dynamically, e.g. bladder diverticulae and vesicoureteric reflux. This is an expensive form of investigation and gives a radiation dose equivalent to a single chest film. Urinary culture, uroflowmetry and videocystography currently are the mainstay of urodynamic investigation, and are collectively the gold standard in urodynamics.

5. *Urethral pressure profilometry.* By definition urinary incontinence only occurs if intravesical pressures exceed those of the outlet resistance, i.e. intraurethral pressure. Microchip technology allows a

pressure profile to be plotted through the bladder, bladder neck and the various parts of the urethra, both at rest and during provocation, e.g. coughing. Urethral instability, a cause of urinary incontinence, may also be studied by this method.

6. *Ultrasound.* This is primarily utilized to image bladder morphology and residual urine volumes. Transvaginal ultrasound may be of use in studying the anatomy of the bladder neck.

7. *Electromyography (EMG).* This is complicated and primarily a tertiary tool to investigate neuropathy and myopathy.

8. *Intravenous urography (IVU) and cystoscopy.* This is useful for investigation of haematuria and frequency and urgency.

Further reading

Versi E, Cardozo L. Urodynamics. In: Studd J, ed. *Progress in Obstetrics and Gynaecology*, Vol. 8. Edinburgh: Churchill Livingstone, 1990; 193–218.

Related topic of interest

Urinary incontinence: incontinence and retention (p. 135)

UTERINE TUMOURS

Benign and malignant tumours of the uterus present at different stages in the patient's reproductive life, with the former tending to be oestrogen dependent while the latter most commonly present in the post-menopausal age group.

Benign tumours

Polyps of glandular origin are commonly associated with hormonal irregularity; typically excess oestrogen stimulation causes hyperplasia of the endometrium. Polyps present with intermenstrual bleeding or menorrhagia. Although usually benign, histological assessment is mandatory to exclude malignancy. Commonly multiple, they may regress with treatment of any underlying hormone imbalance.

Leiomyomata are the commonest benign tumours encountered in gynaecological practice and are discussed separately.

Other benign tumours such as neuromata are extremely rare.

Malignant tumours

The majority of malignant tumours of the body of the uterus are endometrial carcinomata.

Sarcomata may arise in a pre-existing fibroid or, even more rarely, *de novo*.

Secondary deposits do occur in the uterus from primary tumours such as the adjacent cervix, ovary or rectum and distant primaries of breast, kidney and skin (melanoma).

Carcinoma of the endometrium is increasingly common, being the commonest gynaecological cancer in the USA. Over 3000 new cases occur in England and Wales annually, with about 25% of affected women dying of the disease.

Eighty per cent of cases occur in post-menopausal women, the maximum incidence being in the seventh decade. Risk factors include obesity with diabetes and hypertension, unopposed oestrogen therapy, early menarche, late menopause and nulliparity. There is a positive family history in 15% of cases. There is a higher incidence in highly developed countries, which may be related to dietary habits.

Adenocarcinoma is the commonest histological type; there may be associated squamous metaplasia or frankly malignant squamous cells as a coexistent feature.

Spread is directly to adjacent organs or via lymphatics to pelvic or para-aortic nodes, depending on the site of the primary within the uterine cavity. Bloodstream spread to lungs, liver, bone, brain and adrenals is a relatively rare and late event.

The prognosis depends on the stage of the tumour, staging being performed at operation, and taking into account the histological grade of the tumour.

Diagnosis is historically by formal curettage under general anaesthesia at the same time as clinical staging. Less invasive methods of diagnosis, without the need for general anaesthesia, such as endometrial sampling, outpatient hysteroscopy and vaginal ultrasound, either alone or in combination are preferable.

Treatment of early-stage disease is by total abdominal hysterectomy and bilateral salpingo-oophorectomy, pelvic and para aortic lymphaderectomy is advocated, particularly in cases where there is deep myometrial invasion or a high grade tumour. Cervical involvement is treated by radical hysterectomy.

Adjuvant radiotherapy is given for stage 1 disease with deep myometrial involvement, more advanced local disease, high-grade tumour or positive lymph nodes.

For late-stage disease radiotherapy to the pelvis, either pre- or post-operatively, is the mainstay of treatment, with the place of systemic therapy, either hormonal manipulation or cytotoxic chemotherapy, awaiting the results of further evaluation.

Recurrent disease, if confined to the pelvis, may be treated by radiotherapy, if feasible, or radical surgery, including pelvic exenteration where distant spread has been actively excluded. Treatment of extrapelvic disease is by hormones or chemotherapy, both modalities associated with limited survival.

Further reading

Oram D. Management of cancer of the uterine corpus. In: Shepherd JH, Monaghan JM, eds. *Clinical Gynaecological Oncology*, 2nd edn. Oxford: Blackwell Scientific Publications, 1990; 115–39.

Whitfield CR. Benign tumours of the uterus. In: Whitfield CR, ed. *Dewhurst's Textbook of Obstetrics and Gynaecology for Postgraduates*, 4th edn. Oxford: Blackwell Scientific Publications, 1986; 726–32.

Related topics of interest

Cancer of the cervix (p. 16)
Fibroids (p. 35)
Intermenstrual, post-coital and post-menopausal bleeding (p. 65)
Radiotherapy (p. 119)

VAGINAL DISCHARGE

Vaginal discharge is very common. The secretions from the vagina come from several sources, including the vulva, Bartholin's glands, Skene's glands, cervical mucus and endometrial and tubal fluids.

Chemistry

The amount (cervical mucus is the biggest component) and nature of the secretions vary with the menstrual cycle, (premenstrual pH rises to 5.5, pH 3.8–4.2 at ovulation, rises again to 6.5–7.5 during menstruation, post-menopausally pH 6.5) and age. The fluid is acid due to high lactic acid levels and the acidity is influenced by glycogen and lactobacilli, being maximal at birth and ovulation and minimal during childhood and post-menopausally. The menarche and associated oestrogen changes lead to vaginal recolonization with lactobacilli. The vagina also contains many microbes, including staphylococci, streptococci, coliforms and diphtheroids.

Defences

The proximity of the external environment, the urethra and the anus are exacerbating factors, as is sexual activity. The labia form a natural barrier to invasion by pathogens, and the vulval secretions are bacteriostatic. The apposition of the vaginal walls, the acidity, the lack of glands and the normal flora are protective. The cervical mucus contains bacterostatic substances. These may be altered by menstruation (absent mucus, changed pH, menstrual products) and the puerperium (changed pH, low oestrogen levels and friable epithelium, lochial flow).

Diagnosis

(a) History and examination – speculum and inspection.
(b) Cervical cytology and test for pH.
(c) Wet preparation smears, with microscopy.

- Normal saline.
- 10% KOH.

(d) Swabs for culture.
(e) Colposcopy.

Paediatric

See Paediatric gynaecology.

Reproductive years	Mucorrhoea, or excess cervical mucus, is seen in 10% of women, often in association with an ectropion or adenosis. Cervical cryocautery will usually cure it if the cervix is normal to cytology and/or colposcopy. Bacterial discharges are frequent, including *Neisseria gonorrhoea, Gardnerella vaginalis, Treponema pallidum* and *Trichomonas vaginalis.* Each has specific features on history, examination and culture and should respond to standard antibiotic regimens. Sexually acquired infections may require follow-up contact tracing and/or genito-urinary medicine involvement. Viral infections are often chronic, recurring with low-grade virulence, and may be very resistant to treatment. They include genital herpes and condyloma acuminata. Chlamydial disease is generally sexually acquired, may be asymptomatic, and is linked with pelvic infection and tubal destruction, neonatal infection and non-specific urethritis. Tetracyclines are the drugs of choice, with erythromycin being reserved for the pregnant woman. The fungal infections, primarily candidal, are a very common source of vaginal discharge, vaginitis and dyspareunia in young women. Antibiotics, pregnancy, diabetes and immunosuppression are exacerbating factors. A complete course of antifungal medication should be standard, along with treatment of the partner if sexually linked. Resistant disease may respond to oral fluconazole, rather than the more commonly prescribed vaginal pessaries. It is contraindicated in pregnancy. Local potions and bath additives are not recommended and loose cotton underwear is.
Post-menopausal	Atrophy of the lower genital tract secondary to ovarian failure and diminished oestrogen levels is predisposing to inflammation of the vagina and vulva. The post-menopausal years mimic those of the young girl and the breast-feeding mother in vaginal physiological terms. Atrophy may present with pain, dyspareunia, discharge, spotting or bleeding. Hysteroscopy and curettage is mandatory in any with a history of any form of bleeding to exclude malignancy. Treatment is in the form of topical or systemic oestrogens.

Further reading

Emens, JM. The diagnosis and treatment of vaginitis and vaginal discharge. In: Studd J, ed. *Progress in Obstetrics and Gynaecology*, Vol. 3. Edinburgh: Churchill Livingstone, 1988; 213–30.

Related topics of interest

VAGINAL TUMOURS

If cysts of embryological origin are excluded then benign tumours of the vagina are rare. Likewise primary malignant tumours of the vagina have a lower incidence than cervix and corpus uteri, ovary and vulva.

The vagina is the site of origin of sarcoma botryoides in young children and of clear cell carcinoma in young women whose mothers were given exogenous oestrogens in pregnancy.

Benign tumours

These may present as a lump or with dyspareunia. Rarely they may be diagnosed in labour and can present at routine examinations.

Granulomata may occur as a result of previous obstetric injury, as can implantation dermoids. Other tumours include adenomata arising from Gartner's duct and fibromata and lipomata from the subepithelial layers.

Malignant tumours

Over 90% of primary malignancies of the vagina are squamous carcinoma. They constitute 1–2% of genital malignancies. This may underestimate the true incidence as large extensive lesions may be classified as cervical or vulval in origin.

The peak incidence is in the sixth and seventh decades, and predisposing factors include: (i) a history of CIN, particularly if hysterectomy has been performed, with cancer at the vault suture line a particularly difficult management problem; (ii) irritation due to procidentia; a ring pessary or prolapse; chronic infection; previous radiotherapy.

The tumour appears as a lump or an ulcerative mass, the squamous cells exhibiting varying degrees of differentiation, occasionally with keratin whorls.

Spread is direct to adjacent tissues or by lymphatic permeation or embolization. The nodal groups involved depend on the site of the tumour, common sites being the posterior upper third, with spread to pelvic nodes, and the anterior lower third, with spread to both inguinal and pelvic nodes.

1. Clinical features. These patients present with abnormal bleeding, occasionally vaginal discharge and rarely with pain. Diagnosis may be as an incidental finding at a routine examination.

Accurate staging is crucial in the treatment of the disease, and examination under anaesthesia with cystoscopy and sigmoidoscopy, taking appropriate biopsies, is performed.

2. Treatment. Most centres treat all cases with radiotherapy. Better results may be achieved with radical surgery for stage I disease in centres with the necessary expertise.

Overall survival is of the order of:

- 75% 5-year survival in stage I.
- 40–50% in stage II.
- 30% in stage III.
- 0–20% in stage IV (these figures vary as reported series are small).

Surgery is reserved in most centres for recurrent or resistant disease. Some patients survive long term after radical surgery, often pelvic exenteration being necessary.

Rare vaginal malignant tumours

1. Sarcoma botryoides. An embryonal rhabdomyosarcoma arising in the vagina. It is a tumour of childhood, arising at a mean age of 2 years. It presents with bleeding or the appearance of a bloody grape-like mass at the introitus. The treatment of choice is combination chemotherapy and the number of long-term survivors is increasing. Surgery may be necessary as adjunct treatment.

2. Clear cell adenocarcinoma. An association has been found between the development of clear cell carcinoma of the vagina in young women and intake of diethylstilboestrol by their mothers during pregnancy. Histological features are of typical large cells with clear cytoplasm and 'hobnail' nuclei.

Over 500 cases have been reported worldwide since the association was first described in Boston, USA, in 1970, by Herbst and Scully.

Local treatment leads to a high incidence of recurrence, therefore radical surgery or radiotherapy is the main treatment modality.

3. *Malignant melanoma*. This tumour constitutes 1% of vaginal cancers. As with melanoma elsewhere, the prognosis depends on the depth of the lesion, with wide local excision being curative for very superficial lesions, but deeper invasion carrying a very poor prognosis.

Further reading

Monaghan JM. The presentation and management of cancer of the vagina. In: Shepherd JH, Monaghan JM, eds. *Clinical Gynaecological Oncology*, 2nd edn. Oxford: Blackwell Scientific Publications, 1990; 168–87.
Tindall VR. Tumours of the vagina. In: Tindall VR, ed. *Jeffcoate's Principles of Gynaecology*, 5th edn. London: Butterworths, 1987; 389–94.

Related topics of interest

Cancer of the cervix (p. 16)
Paediatric gynaecology (p. 93)
Radiotherapy (p. 119)
Vulva (p. 151)

VULVA

Disorders of the vulva are divided into neoplastic and non-neoplastic although these may co-exist. The latter comprise lichen sclerosus with squamous cell hyperplasia and other dermatoses.

Lichen sclerosus

This is a term to describe a specific inflammatory process of unknown aetiology. Features include the presence of a subepidermal inflammatory cell infiltrate with hyalinization of the epithelium. There is usually thinning of the epithelial layer with loss of rete ridges. At the extreme of the spectrum of this disorder the rete ridges may be elongated when the term squamous cell hyperplasia is used. Lichen sclerosus is often found in association with VIN, although opinion is divided as to whether lichen sclerosus is a premalignant condition.

Diagnosis

The skin may be red or white, flattened or raised, and there may be associated fissuring and ulceration. Some features may be due to scratching that the intense pruritis provokes. Diagnosis is confirmed by skin biopsy, usually under local anaesthesia as an outpatient procedure.

Treatment

The best response is obtained by topical therapy with Clobetasol propionate cream 0.05%. This is applied sparingly twice a day for 3 months in the first instance. Surgery has no place in management although procedures such as skinning vulvectomy are described.

Neoplastic disorders

Vulval intraepithelial neoplasia (VIN)

Cellular atypia confined to the vulval skin (VIN) is associated with infection by oncogenic strains of human papilloma virus (HPV). The skin may be thickened and pruritis is often a feature although patients may be asymptomatic. Diagnosis is by biopsy of affected areas which may be visualized colposcopically after application of 5% acetic acid at least 5 minutes prior to colposcopy. VIN is frequently an incidental finding in association with lichen sclerosus.

Treatment is by surgical excision or laser vapourization although the latter modality is associated with a higher recurrence rate. Progression to invasive cancer is reported although less common than the equivalent process on the cervix. It may be reasonable to keep the area under close surveillance in the asymptomatic patient due to the cosmetic effect of frequent excisions.

Vulval cancer

There are approximately 800 new cases and over 400 deaths from this disease in England and Wales per annum. Although predominantly a disease of elderly women, it has rarely been reported in teenagers and occurs not infrequently in women in their 20s and 30s. Squamous carcinoma is the commonest histological type (85% of cases), with melanoma (10%) and other rarities making up the remainder.

Patients usually present with an ulcer or lump which may be bleeding or secondarily infected. There may be a history of VIN or lichen sclerosus. Diagnosis is confirmed by biopsy. Staging is clinical relating to tumour size, site and presence of lymphatic spread.

Treatment

This tumour spreads to the inguinal lymph nodes. Standard treatment is triple incision vulvectomy and bilateral groin node dissection. Small lateral lesions may be treated by wide local excision and unilateral groin node dissection. Large tumours invading adjacent organs may require more radical surgery, which may be appropriate as a palliative measure even in frail, elderly patients. The key is individualization of management. Adjuvant radiotherapy is utilized if there are groin node metastases.

Microinvasion

When the depth of invasion of small tumours is reported as less than 1 mm beneath the basement membrane then local excision is adequate therapy. Groin node dissection is indicated for deeper invasion.

Complications

Wound breakdown and infection are common problems and lead to prolonged hospitalization. Surgical technique and post-operative nursing are of prime importance.

Lymphoedema is an effect of node dissection and may lead to distressing chronic swelling of the lower limbs. This is minimized by suction drainage of groin wounds, early mobilization and physiotherapy (limb elevation and massage) and support hosiery.

Further reading

Gleeson NC. The management of vulval dystrophy. In: Bonnar J, ed. *Recent Advances in Obstetrics and Gynaecology,* Vol. 19. Edinburgh: Churchill Livingstone, 1995; 191–200.

Monaghan JM. The management of carcinoma of the vulva. In: Shepherd JH, Monaghan JM, eds. *Clinical Gynaecological Oncology*, 2nd edn. Oxford: Blackwell Scientific Publications, 1990; 140–67.

Related topics of interest

ABDOMINAL PAIN IN PREGNANCY

Most women experience pain at some time in a pregnancy. A woman's awareness of her pregnancy may well predispose her to seeking help early on. Pain in pregnancy may be physiological or pathological, pregnancy related or incidental. The management of pain in pregnancy will depend upon the diagnosis, and in most cases will be conservative.

The anatomy of pain

1. *Uterine body.* T10-L1 sensory afferent, with corresponding pain dermatomes being from umbilicus to symphysis, laterally to the iliac crests and posteriorly to lumbar and sacral vertebrae.

2. *Cervix.* As above, plus additional sensory to S2, S3 and S4.

3. *Ovary.* T10 sensory afferent running in the sympathetic chain. Note that the gynaecological sensory nerves overlap other pelvic and abdominal structures, so localization and diagnosis may be difficult.

Pain directly related to pregnancy

First trimester

(a) Abortion related, particularly if septic.
(b) Hydatidiform mole.
(c) Ectopic (prevalence 0.5%), linked with salpingitis, IUCD, previous ectopic pregnancy, tubal or other pelvic surgery.
(d) Ovarian cyst, haemorrhage or torsion.

Second trimester

(a) Abortion related.
(b) Acute urinary retention in association with a retroverted gravid uterus, classically at 12–14 weeks.
(c) Chorioamnionitis or retroplacental haemorrhage secondary to amniocentesis.
(d) So-called 'ligamentous' pain due to stretch of round and broad ligaments, classically at 18–22 weeks.
(e) 'Red degeneration' of a fibroid.

Third trimester

(a) Placental abruption, with or without bleeding.
(b) Pre-eclampsia and eclampsia – particularly of the epigastrium and the right upper quadrant, with hepatic capsule stretch.

(c) Uterine rupture secondary to previous uterine surgery, Caesarean section.
(d) Fetal movements and Braxton-Hicks contractions.
(e) Abdominal distension and flank pain secondary to visceral displacement from the enlarging uterus.

Pain not directly related to pregnancy

Gastrointestinal tract

(a) Gastro-oesophageal reflux, common to most pregnancies.
(b) Constipation, common to most pregnancies.
(c) Haemorrhoids.
(d) Hiatus hernia.
(e) Appendicitis. The diagnosis may be difficult because the appendix site rises with gestation. The frequency is approximately 1:2500 pregnancies.
(f) Peptic ulcer, uncommon.
(g) Gall bladder disease: pregnancy is a cholestatic process.
(h) Pancreatitis: rare but has high mortality (>10%).
(i) Bowel obstruction: uncommon, but may occur after Caesarean section.
(j) Inflammatory bowel disease – may be present in pregnancy.

Renal tract

(a) Urinary tract infection: 5% of pregnant women have asymptomatic bacteriuria.
(b) Pyelonephritis: prevalence approximately 1%, mostly in second and third trimesters.
(c) Renal calculi: uncommon because of physiological dilatation of the renal tract. The frequency is approximately 1:1500 pregnancies.

Incidental causes of pain in pregnancy

(a) Pre-existing musculoskeletal pain, exacerbated by the abnormal carriage of the gravid abdomen.
(b) Hip, leg and pelvic joint pain secondary to the joint laxity of pregnancy and nerve stretch and/or entrapment.
(c) Vascular accidents:

- Rectus sheath haematoma.
- Sickle cell crisis.
- Rarely splenic and aneurysmal rupture.

(d) Malignant pain – may be a new presentation.

(e) Porphyria – uncommon.

Further reading

Setchell M. Abdominal pain in pregnancy. In: Studd J, ed. *Progress in Obstetrics and Gynaecology*, Vol. 6. Edinburgh: Churchill Livingstone, 1987; 87–99.

Related topic of interest

Chronic pelvic pain (p. 19)

ABNORMAL UTERINE FUNCTION IN LABOUR

Uterine function in labour is said to be abnormal if the rate of cervical dilatation falls below the minimum rate accepted by a particular obstetric unit (usually around 1 cm/h), in the absence of cephalopelvic disproportion or cervical dystocia.

Measurement of uterine activity is via an intrauterine pressure transducer, the units of measurement being kPa/15 min. The accepted range for normal uterine contractions is 700–1800 kPa/15 min, corresponding to the 10th and 90th centiles respectively.

Factors involved in generation of intrauterine pressures are the strength and duration of individual contractions and their frequency. Pressures are calculated from the area under the curve generated by each contraction in a 15-min period. This accurately reflects uterine activity provided the baseline tone is normal.

The myometrium acts as a syncytium, with pressure waves generated from the fundus and travelling toward the cervix. Nerve supply is sparse, the stimuli to contraction being largely hormonal and biochemical.

It is suggested that delay in labour is related to an abnormal cervical ripening response which may be better overcome by cervical ripening agents (e.g. relaxin) than by oxytoxic agents, the latter giving rise to fetal distress in this situation.

Problems

1. *Hypotonic uterine activity.* This is the commonest form of abnormal function. Easily overcome by oxytocic stimulation in the majority of cases, this phenomenon is largely confined to primigravidae in the absence of a predisposing cause.

Associated factors include stress (adrenaline in small concentrations markedly inhibits uterine activity), pain (either by increasing stress or by increasing sympathetic activity) and the supine position (for reasons which are unclear).

Various workers have demonstrated a reversal of uterine hypotonicity using agents such as pethidine, epidural analgesia and propranolol or by correcting the supine position.

Reduction in stress levels may indirectly give rise to cervical ripening and subsequent dilation by reducing tension forces on the cervix.

2. *Hypertonic uterine activity.* This is more significant in that the pressure increase can inhibit uterine blood flow and predispose to fetal hypoxia.

Idiopathic hypertonicity is rare, the commonest cause being iatrogenic overstimulation with oxytocic agents, followed by placental abruption.

Occasional hypersensitive reactions occur with prostaglandin administration, associated fetal distress necessitating urgent delivery.

The effect of overstimulation with intravenous oxytocin may be reversed after about 5 min by discontinuing the infusion.

In the presence of fetal distress, prompt reversal of the effect may be achieved with the administration of an intravenous tocolytic agent such as salbutamol. Urgent delivery by Caesarean section may be necessary.

The hypertonicity of abruptio placentae is invariably accompanied by a marked rise in the rate of contractions. Pain is a usual associated symptom.

Management is dictated by the degree of fetal distress and maternal blood loss. Tocolytics are never administered in the presence of an abruption.

Conclusion

Slow labour is commonly due to inefficient uterine contractions, which may be overcome by the use of oxytocic agents. Careful monitoring of patients receiving oxytocic infusions is mandatory to avoid the effects of overstimulation on the uterine blood supply and consequent fetal distress.

Further reading

Gibb DMF, Arulkumaran S. Uterine contractions and the fetus. In: Studd J, ed. *Progress in Obstetrics and Gynaecology*, Vol. 6. Edinburgh: Churchill Livingstone, 1987; 133–53.

Gee H, Olah KS. Failure to progress in labour. In: Studd J, ed. *Progress in Obstetrics and Gynaecology,* Vol. 10. Edinburgh: Churchill Livingstone, 1993; 159–81.

Steer PJ. Abnormal uterine action. In: Turnbull Sir AC, Chamberlain GC, eds. *Obstetrics.* Edinburgh: Churchill Livingstone, 1989; 783–92.

Related topics of interest

AMNIOTIC FLUID EMBOLUS

Amniotic fluid embolism is still a significant cause of maternal mortality, although there has been a slight fall over the last 20 years. It must be suspected in all cases of sudden maternal collapse. It is thought that the amniotic fluid will enter through the endocervical veins or the placental bed, although uterine trauma will also allow for entry of amniotic fluid into the circulation.

Associated factors

1. Maternal. Multiparity, elderly (>25), LSCS, term pregnancy, tumultuous labour, uterine stimulation, uterine manipulation.

2. Fetal. Large baby, intrauterine death, placental abruption, at SROM and/or ARM.

Clinical signs

Can be sudden or dramatic collapse resulting in death or a combination of respiratory distress, cyanosis, cardiovascular collapse, haemorrhage (DIC) and coma.

Treatment

Is initially supportive. Immediate institution of CPR may be necessary with the maintenance clear airway and intubation with immediate cricoid pressure to prevent regurgitation.

100% O_2 should be given and cardiac compression with patient tilted to right may be required.

Monitoring central venous load with careful infusion of FFP and packed red cells when necessary.

Immediate surgical delivery is required if not previously delivered with stimulation of uterine contraction.

Once the patient has been stabilized then they should be transfered to ITU for ventilation.

Discussion

Confidential report into maternal deaths in the United Kingdom in 1996 for the years 1991–1993 reported 128 deaths associated purely with obstetric causes. Of these 10 were due to amniotic fluid embolism.

It is associated with a very high mortality rate of 80%, approximately half occurring at the time of the sudden collapse.

Death usually occurs as a result of cardiorespiratory collapse or disseminated intravascular coagulation.

Diagnosis is very difficult and is often confirmed at post-mortem when amniotic fluid, fetal squames or lanugo are found in the maternal circulation.

There are certain diagnostic pointers such as fetal squames found in maternal sputum and also in blood aspirated from the right atrium, right ventricular strain on ECG and also perihilar infiltrates on chest on chest X-ray.

Lethal amniotic fluid embolism is most commonly associated with small tears in the uterus, cervix, or vagina which have not totally disrupted the wall.

Coagulation failure occurs rapidly but the complete pulmonary shut down is the first sign. This results from amniotic fluid plugging the pulmonary vessels and the subsequent release of vasoactive substances leading to vascular constriction. The coagulation abnormality is attributed to the thromboplastic activity of amniotic fluid.

Further reading

Letsky EL. Coagulation defects in pregnancy. In: Turnbull Sir AC, Chamberlain GC, eds. *Obstetrics.* 1989; 568–9.

Mulder JL. Amniotic fluid embolus: an overview and case report. *American Journal of Obstetrics and Gynaecology*, 1985; **152:** 430–5.

Report on Confidential Enquiries into Maternal Deaths in the United Kingdom 1991–1993.

Related topics of interest

Coagulation and pregnancy (p. 191)

Report on Confidential Enquiry into Maternal Deaths in the United Kingdom 1991–1993 (p. 309)

ANAEMIA IN PREGNANCY

The World Health Organization recommend a minimum haemoglobin level of 11.0 g/dl during pregnancy. The physiological changes during pregnancy predispose to the development of an anaemic state.

Iron-deficiency anaemia

Women have a precarious iron balance status due to continued menstrual loss. During pregnancy this is aggravated by the increased requirements of the extra red cells and the iron requirements of the fetus (manifest mainly at about 32 weeks' gestation and later).

Iron absorption is erratic, absorption of animal haemoglobin and myoglobin of red meat being most efficient and absorption of the inorganic ferric form least efficient.

More sensitive than haemoglobin estimation is the measurement of serum ferritin, and one study has estimated that 82.5% of women with adequate haemoglobin levels at booking are in fact iron deficient by other accepted haematological criteria. This forms the basis for recommending prophylactic iron supplements in pregnancy.

Megaloblastic anaemia

This is much more commonly the result of folate deficiency as vitamin B_{12} stores are usually adequate. Extra folate is required to meet the demands of the fetus and placenta as well as increased requirements of the red cells. The overall frequency in the United Kingdom is about 5%, but this figure is increased if the bone marrow is examined. Folate is present in a wide range of foods, mainly green vegetables, but is rapidly destroyed in cooking. Women of lower social class are more likely to have a folate-deficient diet. Most oral iron supplements in pregnancy also contain folate.

Folate deficiency is implicated in neural tube defects. All women are advised to take preconceptual folic acid supplements: 4 mg to 400 mg daily, depending on the degree of risk.

Folate requirements are increased in patients on anticonvulsant therapy.

Haemoglobinopathies

These anaemias occur as a result of abnormal globin synthesis (sickle cell anaemia) or impaired globin synthesis (thalassaemias).

Sickle cell anaemia

This is caused by abnormal globin structure. There are many variants, the most important of which are HbS and HbC. Homozygous SS or heterozygous SC commonly gives rise to an increased frequency of sickling crises in pregnancy. Heterozygous HbS thalassaemia occurs and is clinically indistinguishable from HbSS.

The mainstay of treatment is supportive therapy, mainly oxygen and analgesia. Diagnosis is by haemoglobin electrophoresis, and antenatal diagnosis is available in early pregnancy for affected couples.

Thalassaemia

One gene from each parent specifies production of the beta-globin chain, while two genes from each parent specify the alpha-chain.

Beta-thalassaemia minor occurs when one defective gene is inherited and is usually asymptomatic until anaemia develops in pregnancy when oral iron and folate are required. Beta-thalassaemia major, the homozygous condition, gives rise to a severe anaemia, uniformly fatal before the advent of safe blood transfusion. These patients are extremely unlikely to become pregnant, antenatal diagnosis in the heterozygote being the main concern.

Alpha-thalassaemia major, with no alpha-chains formed, is incompatible with life.

Degrees of alpha-thalassaemia occur depending on whether one, two or three defective genes are inherited. HbH occurs when only one gene producing alpha-chains is present and is associated with severe anaemia and high folate requirements. These patients are at risk of an alpha-thalassaemia hydrops (a fetus with alpha-thalassaemia major), which is associated with life-threatening pre-eclampsia.

Again, antenatal diagnosis is of particular importance in this group of patients.

Further reading

Letsky EA. Blood volume, haematinics, anaemia. In: De Swiet M, ed. *Medical Disorders in Obstetric Practice*. Oxford: Blackwell Scientific Publications, 1989; 48–103.

Related topics of interest

Hydrops fetalis (p. 223)
Physiology of pregnancy (p. 260)
Prenatal diagnosis (p. 281)

ANALGESIA / ANAESTHESIA IN LABOUR

Points to be covered

(a) Non-pharmacological methods of pain relief.
(b) Inhalational analgesics.
(c) Narcotic analgesics.
(d) Epidural analgesia (including local anaesthetics).
(e) General anaesthesia.

Non-pharmacological

A friendly atmosphere, homely surroundings, patient education and a caring midwife all decrease the need for analgesia in labour.

Hypnosis, acupuncture, and more recently aromatherapy have all been used to some effect.

The most common method is transcutaneous electrical nerve stimulation (TENS). Electrodes are placed over the posterior primary rami of T10-L1 and S2-4 and a current passed between them. The level of current can be increased during a contraction. TENS probably works by stimulating large sensory fibres which will inturn inhibit transmitter release in the pain pathways (Melzack and Wall Gate Theory).

Inhalational analgesia

First used by Queen Victoria when chloroform was administered to her by John Snow.

Nitrous oxide is now the single most widely used inhalational analgesic in the UK.

Other volatile agents such as enflurane and isoflurane have all been investigated but show little advantage over nitrous oxide.

Entonox, the 50:50 mix of N_2O and O_2 that is now commonly used, is a poor analgesic. The method involves the patient hyperventilating trying to obtain pain relief that rapidly wears off. This can result in hypocapnia and even tetany. Theoretically even fetal hypoxia can result due to the Bohr effect and uterine vasoconstriction, but this is offset by the 50% O_2 in entonox. Nausea, light-headedness, and lack of pain relief are reasons for discontinuing the use of inhalational analgesia.

Narcotic analgesics

Pethidine may be given by midwives for pain relief in labour. It is a powerful sedative, is associated with a high incidence of nausea and vomiting and a 20% reduction in pain score.

Inappropriate in fulminating pre-eclampsia as its metabolite has convulsant properties.

The most serious side effect of the use of opiod analgesics during labour is a delay in gastric emptying, therefore the routine use of ranitidine is encouraged whenever opioids are administered.

Respiratory depression in the newborn is greatest when the administration is within an hour of birth. Naloxone may counteract this problem.

Patient controlled analgesia has been used, but infants delivered to women treated with PCA required more naloxone, so the method has not been widely used. Partial opioid agonists such as pentazocine, meptazinol and nalbuphine have all been used, but have not replaced pethidine as the first choice drug.

Epidural analgesia

Contraindications to an epidural are maternal refusal, coagulopathy, sepsis and thrombocytopenia.

Common indications are as follows:

- *Pain relief.*
- *Breech presentation.*
- *Multiple pregnancy.*
- *Rotational forceps delivery.*
- *Caesarean sections.*
- *Pre-eclampsia.*
- *Previous LSCS.*
- *Premature labour.*
- *Prolonged labour and the need for oxytocin.*
- *Cardiovascular and respiratory disease.* Under certain circumstances it may be desirable to avoid the stress of a painful labour and risk of a GA should operative delivery be necessary.

Complications occur and appear to be related to the experience of the anaesthetist. The incidence of accidental dural puncture is 1–2%. A bloody tap can also occur.

Aspiration of the catheter prior to top-up is important to prevent administration of the local anaesthetic agent into a vein or the CSF.

If a total spinal anaesthetic occurs then the woman is at risk of rapidly rising numbness, dyspnoea, unconsciousness, and cardiorespiratory collapse. Prompt resuscitation must therefore be available.

Post dural puncture headaches are common occurring within 1–2 days and lasting for several weeks, the prevalence being approximately 70%.

Continuous infusion techniques and the use of spinal opioids have improved the efficacy of epidurals.

There is no conclusive evidence that a well managed epidural increases the forceps rate, or that withholding epidural top-up as second stage approaches increases the chance of a normal delivery.

There is no demonstrable association between epidural analgesia in labour and new post partum headache.

General anaesthesia

This is still a significant cause of maternal morbidity and mortality and appears to be associated with inexperienced anaesthetists with a poor standard of help available.

Aspiration of gastric contents must be prevented. Oral ranitidine (45 minutes needed for effect) and the non-particulate antacid sodium citrate are given. Cricoid pressure is applied at induction.

Aorta-caval compression during anaesthesia is minimized by the use of left lateral tilt of the patient.

Mendelson's syndrome (aspiration pneumonitis) and failure of intubation are the two greatest risks of a general anaesthetic during pregnancy.

Further reading

Reynolds F. Epidural analgesia in obstetrics. Pros and cons for mother and baby. *British Medical Journal*, 1989; **299:** 751–2 (Editorial).

Moir DD, Thorburn J. Obstetric anaesthesia and analgesia. 1986; 3rd edn. London: Balliere Tindall.

Reynolds F. Dural puncture and headache. *British Medical Journal,* 1993, **306:** 874–5.

Russel R, Reynolds F. Back pain, pregnancy and childbirth. *British Medical Journal,* 1997, **314:** 1062–3.

Related topics of interest

ANATOMY OF THE FEMALE PELVIS, THE FETAL SKULL AND THE FETAL CIRCULATION

The *female bony pelvis* is formed by the union of the sacrum and coccyx with the ilium, the ischium and the pubis. Posteriorly, this union is effected by the sacroiliac ligaments supporting the sacroiliac joints and the sacral and coccygeal vertebrae divided by the intervertebral discs; anteriorly the union is effected by the symphysis pubis. The important bony landmarks are the inlet of the true pelvis, the outlet of the true pelvis, the subpubic arch and the ischial spines. The inlet (AP inlet) is represented by a straight line drawn from the anterior border of the sacral promontory to the posterior border of the upper symphysis pubis, and is bordered laterally by the iliopectineal lines. The outlet (AP outlet) is represented by a straight line drawn from the lower anterior border of the sacrum to the lower posterior border of the symphysis pubis, and is bordered laterally along the pubic rami to the ischial tuberosities, the ischial spines and the lower anterior border of the sacrum. The AP inlet and outlet, at radiological pelvimetry, should be at least 11.5 cm if the pelvis is to be considered adequate. In the anatomical position an angle of 135° (the angle of inclination) exists between the plane of the pelvic inlet and a vertical line drawn through the spine. The subpubic arch is important in that as it diminishes it reduces the diameter of the outlet. The ischial spines are a vital obstetric landmark denoting the station of the presenting part and the site of the pudendal nerve and vessels. The basic shape of the bony pelvis is gynaecoid, with android, platypelloid and anthropoid being variations denoted by different diameters.

The *soft tissue anatomy of the pelvic floor* is dominated by the pair of symmetrical, striated muscles known as the levator ani or pelvic diaphragm. Levator ani is divided into three components: the pubococcygeus (itself divided into an anterior puborectalis and a posterior part), the ileococcygeus and a smaller coccygeus. The nerve supply is twofold: pudendal from the anterior primary rami of S2, S3 and S4 and direct from the motor roots of S3 and S4. The muscle is in continuous activity, even in a sleep state, and is composed of fast- and slow-twitch fibres to cope with continence, parturition, micturition and defecation. The muscle floor is defective in the midline to allow the passage of the urethra, the vagina, the rectum and anal canal. The female urethra is 4 cm long and runs from the bladder, anteroinferiorly, to emerge at the external meatus between the origins of pubococcygeus. The urethra is supplied by the pudendal nerve, as is the external anal sphincter. The fascia of the pelvic floor is vital to its integrity, providing via its attachment to the pelvic brim and the muscle a framework for function. It is condensed in areas to form the uterosacral, transverse cervical and pubourethral ligaments. The bladder base is supported by the pubovesical fascia, whilst posterior to the uterus lie the musculofascial structures of the perineal body, the anal canal and the post-anal plate. The suspensory ligaments of the rectum are provided by condensations of the presacral fascia.

The *fetal skull* develops from mesenchyme around the developing brain, and is in two parts: the *neurocranium,* or protective case for the brain, and the *viscerocranium,* or main jaw skeleton. Each of these develops via cartilaginous and membranous stages. The membranous neurocranium forms the cranial vault. In fetal and infant life the skull flat bones are separated by dense connective tissue membranes or fibrous joints, with two or more sutures meeting at fibrous areas known as fontanelles. The two main fontanelles are the diamond-shaped anterior, at the junction of the frontal, sagittal and two lateral coronal sutures, and the triangular posterior, at the junction of the sagittal and two oblique lambdoid sutures. The plasticity of the fetal skull bones, in conjunction with their loose suture and fontanelle connections, enables the skull to undergo shape changes or moulding during labour and delivery. A knowledge of fetal skull anatomy is essential to enable a diagnosis of malposition to be made in a labour with a cephalic presentation.

The fetal circulation is dependent upon precocious development to meet the needs of nutrient acquisition for rapid growth and disposal of waste products (hence blood is circulating by the end of the third embryonic week) and can be adapted at delivery to serve extrauterine life. The sequential route of a unit of blood in the fetal circulation is as follows:

Placenta $\Rightarrow$ single umbilical vein (80% saturation) $\Rightarrow$ hepatic sinusoids (50% of flow) and ductus venosus (50% of flow) (liver bypass) $\Rightarrow$ IVC $\Rightarrow$ right atrium (the saturation drops because of mixing with deoxygenated blood from the lower limbs, abdomen and pelvis) $\Rightarrow$ crista dividens (diverts blood through the foramen ovale) $\Rightarrow$ left atrium (there is a further small drop in saturation here as a result of mixing with deoxygenated blood returning from the fetal pulmonary veins) $\Rightarrow$ left ventricle $\Rightarrow$ ascending aorta (hence the heart, head and neck and upper limbs receive well-oygenated blood). A small amount of IVC blood remains in the right atrium and is mixed with deoxygenated blood from the superior vena cava (SVC) and coronary sinus $\Rightarrow$ right ventricle $\Rightarrow$ pulmonary trunk $\Rightarrow$ ductus arteriosus $\Rightarrow$ aorta (pulmonary artery blood flow is low because of very high pulmonary vascular resistance). Fifty-eight per cent of the saturated blood in the descending aorta passes into the two umbilical arteries for return to the placenta.

At birth thoracic compression, change in temperature, tactile stimuli, drop in pH and rise in pCO_2 lead to initiation of respiration and adult circulation. Lung aeration causes a marked drop in pulmonary vascular resistance and increases in pulmonary blood flow and left atrial pressure. Placental occlusion causes a fall in the blood pressure of the IVC and right atrium, which leads to functional closure of the foramen ovale. The ductus arteriosus and umbilical arteries constrict at birth. The adult derivatives of these important structures are:

- Umbilical vein = ligamentum teres.

- Ductus venosus = ligamentum venosum.
- Foramen ovale = fossa ovalis.
- Ductus arteriosus = ligamentum arteriosum.
- Umbilical arteries = medial umbilical ligaments and superior vesical arteries.

Further reading

Moore KL. *The Developing Human,* 2nd edn. Philadelphia: WB Saunders, 1977.

Related topic of interest

Neonatology (p. 251)

ANTEPARTUM HAEMORRHAGE

The definition of an APH (antepartum haemorrhage) is bleeding (>15 ml) from the genital tract after 24 weeks and prior to delivery of the infant.

20% of women will bleed at some time in their pregnancy; in 4% this will occur in the third trimester.

Bleeding can occur from an abnormally situated placenta (praevia), a normally situated placenta (abruption) and bleeding from other sites (incidental).

Placenta praevia

Placenta is partly or wholly inserted in the lower uterine segment at or after 28 weeks gestation, prior to 28 weeks the placenta is termed low-lying. It is divided into four grades by the Dewhurst classification:

I: placenta just encroaches into lower segment.
II: placenta reaches the margin of the cervical os.
III: placenta covers the os but not at full dilatation.
IV: placenta covers the cervical os completely (centric).

The higher the grade, the higher the maternal and fetal morbidity and mortality.

The frequency of placenta praevia is between 0.4–0.8%. Associated factors include twins, age, multiparity, cigarette smoking, D&C and previous Caesarean section. The latter is also associated with increased incidence of placenta accreta.

Perinatal mortality rates as high as 81/1000 have been reported, with a 22% incidence of RDS.

Classically it presents with painless bleeding around 35 weeks; clinically there is a high presenting part or malpresentation with the diagnosis confirmed by ultrasound or MRI. Vaginal examination is totally contraindicated. Thirty four per cent of women with placenta praevia have no history of haemorrhage antenatally.

Management
The asymptomatic patient does not necessarily require total inpatient care, however it is important to perform serial scanning in the third trimester to check on growth and placental site.

When a patient is admitted bleeding then resuscitation of the patient should be paramount, intravenous access, cross match 4-units of blood (which should then be always available) and admit to hospital.

Fetal viability must be confirmed and then monitored regularly with CTG and USS.

Expectant management should be followed postponing delivery until 37 weeks unless earlier intervention is indicated for fetal or maternal reasons.

Delivery is by Caesarean section normally under GA for grade II (where necessary), III or IV placenta praevia, with the most senior obstetrician available performing the operation. There is a well known association with PPH.

Placental abruption

Placental attachment to the uterine wall is disrupted by haemorrhage. Occurs in 1% of pregnancies. It has a recurrence rate of about 6%.

Associated factors include a raised AFP, trauma to the abdomen, maternal hypertension, cigarette smoking, sudden uterine decompression and presence of the lupus anticoagulant, polyhydramnios and seat belt injuries.

It classically presents as bleeding, severe pain and premature labour. The vaginal bleeding may be minimal in comparison to the abruption – the so called Couvelaire uterus. It is also associated with intrauterine death. In severe abruption a coagulopathy can occur.

Diagnosis is usually clinical although confirmation may be sought with an USS.

Management
Ascertaining fetal viability along with resuscitation of the patient are again of paramount importance. If fetal demise has occurred then cross-matching 4-units of blood and a clotting screen should be performed.

If minor abruption is confirmed clinically and with confirmatory CTG and USS evidence then expectant management should be followed. If a major abruption is diagnosed and the fetus is viable then immediate delivery should occur by LSCS. In major abruption (with or without IUD) it is important to involve an experienced anaesthetist in fluid balance, monitoring and replacement and a haematologist for discussion about abnormal coagulation. Careful monitoring of the coagulation state (prevention DIC) is very important.

Other sites

Lower genital tract e.g. Cervical polyps, trauma. Coagulation defects e.g. Von-Willebrand's, Warfarin.

Vasa-praevia is where a placental blood vessel lies in front of the presenting part of the fetus – usually due to a velomentous insertion of the cord into the placenta.

Bleeding from this will cause vaginal bleeding but also exsanguination of the fetus. Fetal haemoglobin can be checked for by using NaOH or by performing a Kleihauer test.

Rarely carcinoma of the cervix can present as an APH.

Further reading

Baron SL. Antepartum haemorrhage. In: Turnbull Sir AC, Chamberlain GC, eds. *Obstetrics.* Edinburgh: Churchill Livingstone, 1990; **32:** 469–82.

Egley C, Cefalo RC. Abruptio placenta. In: Studd J, ed. *Progress in Obstetrics and Gynaecology,* 5th edn. Edinburgh: Churchill Livingstone, 1984; 108–20.

Penna LK, Pearce JM. Placenta praevia. In: Studd J, ed. *Progress in Obstetrics and Gynaecology*, 1994; **11:** 161–81.

Related topics of interest

BIOPHYSICAL PROFILE – ASSESSING THE AT RISK FETUS

The biophysical profile (BPP) is a means of assessing fetal well-being and predicting the at-risk fetus, using five parameters;

(a) Fetal breathing movements: determined via USS.
(b) Gross body movements: determined via USS.
(c) Fetal tone: determined via USS.
(d) Qualitative amniotic fluid volume: determined via USS.
(e) Reactive fetal heart rate (non-stress test):   determined via cardiotocography.

Discussion

Each parameter scores 0 or 2 with the maximum being 10. Its aim is to predict the at risk fetus. The frequency of monitoring is dependent upon gestation and the BPP score, but in general if the score is satisfactory, for example >6, then weekly or twice weekly assessment will be adequate.

The commonest causes of perinatal death are asphyxia (60%), congenital anomalies (25%) and prematurity (15%). Fetal asphyxia will cause central nervous system depression and resultant losses or alterations to the fetal biophysical activities under direct CNS control. Thus an acute hypoxaemic episode will result in loss of fetal breathing, fetal flexor tone and fetal heart rate accelerations. Chronic hypoxaemia is manifest with oligohydramnios (normal amniotic fluid volumes range between 2–8 cm, with oligohydramnios being <2 cm and polyhydramnios being >8 cm) and extrinsic growth failure. The advantage of a BPP is that it encompasses simultaneous measurement of both acute and chronic indices of fetal asphyxia. The BPP has validity, in gestational age terms, from the time of fetal viability, i.e. 24 weeks. In addition to BPP criteria, USS of the at risk fetus is useful in predicting estimated fetal weight (EFW) and when performed serially will give a trend in fetal growth, which can then be compared to singleton fetus nomograms and centile curves.

The use of computerized antenatal cardiotocography, as developed by Dawes and Redman, has given another parameter to fetal assessment by calculating the mean range; a computed assessment of fetal heart rate variability. The normal range is >30, suspicion about the fetus being at risk with a score of 20–30 and a definite at risk fetus with a score <20.

The use of biophysical profile scoring in the management of high risk pregnancies has been extensively studied in Canada by Manning and his colleagues. They have found that perinatal mortality could be reduced to 5.06/1000 total births, compared to an untested high risk population where it was 65/1000. The false negative rate, i.e. stillbirth within one week of a normal test result, was 0.8/1000. This compares very well with the non-stress CTG that can give a false negative rate of up to 3/1000. Analysis of the outcome of high risk fetuses assessed by computerized mean range scoring are awaited with interest. The positive predictive accuracy of an abnormal BPP (<4) is confirmed, with the perinatal mortality rising inversely with the BPP score e.g. 22/1000 when 4, rising to 187/1000 with a score of 0.

Non-reactive CTG and loss of fetal breathing movements are the first manifestations of fetal acidosis. In advanced acidaemia fetal tone and movements are compromised. Reduced liquor volume is a chronic sign.

There is significant relationship between BPP and fetal acid base status shown by blood taken at cordocentesis or following Caesarean section.

The use of Doppler flow studies of cord blood flow between placenta and fetus have been used successfully. The initial measurement made is the resistance index. However, the two most important findings are absent end-diastolic flow or reversed end-diastolic flow, both of which may indicate an at risk fetus and warrant delivery.

Further reading

Baskett TF. The fetal biophysical profile. In: Studd J, ed. *Progress in Obstetrics and Gynaecology*, Volume 7. 1989; **9:** 145–59.

Dawes GS, Houghton RS, Redman CWG *et al.* Pattern of the normal human fetal heart rate. *British Journal of Obstetrics and Gynaecology*, 1982; **89:** 276–84.

Manning FA, Meticoglou S, Harman C. Fetal assessment by biophysical methods: Ultrasound. In: Turnbull Sir AC, Chamberlain GC, eds. *Obstetrics.* Edinburgh: Churchill Livingstone, 1991; **27**: 383–98.

Related topics of interest

Monitoring in labour (p. 245)
Intrauterine growth retardation (p. 241)

BREECH

The incidence of breech presentation varies inversely with gestation, 16% at 32 weeks, 7% at 38 weeks and falling finally to 3–4% at 40 weeks.

The majority of breech presentations at term are thought to have had a cornual implantation of the placenta.

The mechanism of breech labour involves the bitrochanteric diameter (9.25 cm) entering the pelvis in the transverse plane, rotating in the mid pelvis and presenting at the pelvic outlet in the anterior–posterior diameter.

There are three types of breech presentation:

(a) Extended breech (65%).
(b) Flexed breech (25%).
(c) Footling breech (10%).

Associated factors

1. Fetal. Extended legs preventing spontaneous version, fetal anomaly, e.g. hydrocephalus, anencephaly, cystic hygroma; prematurity and twins.

2. Maternal. Uterine anomaly, placenta praevia, pelvic tumours, e.g. ovarian cyst, cervical fibroid; and polyhydramnios.

Management of the persistent breech presentation is important and a number of steps should be followed prior to allowing a vaginal delivery to occur. In the case of a footling breech, Caesarean section is always advised.

Ultrasound scanning

This should be performed to exclude fetal abnormality; localize the placenta, confirm fetal presentation, estimation of fetal weight is important because if the estimated fetal weight is between 3500–3700 g or greater then an elective Caesarean section should be considered, and finally the attitude of the fetal head is important as extension of the fetal head (so called star gazing) is a contraindication to vaginal delivery. It must be remembered that there may be large errors in estimating fetal weight, possibly more so with breech presentation than cephalic.

Pelvimetry

The efficacy of X-ray pelvimetry is controversial and it carries risks, however it is becoming a necessary medico-legal event.

There are three current methods in use, erect lateral X-ray of the pelvis, CT scan of the pelvis and finally the use of MRI has been used. Whatever measure is used the obstetrician must see the pictures himself to measure the inlet and outlet (both must be >11.5 cm), and to assess the sacral curve, because a 'flat' sacrum is not ideal for a vaginal delivery.

Discussion

These criteria will result in a 25% LSCS rate. Even then it is crucial to watch the progress of the selected patients in labour. Augmentation with syntocinon is contentious. Use of syntocinon in the first stage is well recognized, whereas its use later in the second stage to drive a too big breech into the pelvis is contraindicated.

Labour should progress at least at a rate of 1 cm/h during first stage. After allowing 1 hour for descent in second stage, if the infant has not delivered within 1 hour of active pushing, then an LSCS should be performed, as it is likely that either the baby is bigger than first thought or the pelvis is smaller than thought.

At the time of membrane rupture vaginal examination is imperative to exclude cord prolapse and confirm whether the breech is flexed or not. Fetal monitoring is imperative. Breech extraction should *never* be performed in the singleton, but assisted breech delivery should be. Episiotomy should be performed when the fetal anus has appeared at the vulva. Hyperextension of the neck during delivery should be prevented as this can cause compression of the vertebral arteries and subsequent necrosis of the spinal cord. The sole indication for symphysiotomy is failure of the head to engage; however with proper predelivery assessment the technique will never be necessary.

Management of the preterm breech in labour is important as the incidence of a breech presentation prior to 37 weeks is 15%. If vaginal delivery is decided upon then an epidural anaesthetic is advisable to prevent the mother pushing when the cervix is not fully dilated and also to relax the pelvic floor. Some authorities advocate a caul delivery, i.e. within the complete amniotic sac. As in all cases, the infant must be handled carefully and a paediatrician must be present.

There is a risk of head entrapment with an undilated cervix. Tocolytics may be useful. Flexion of the head and turning the baby into the transverse can sometimes help, and as a final resort, releasing incisions in the cervix at 4 and 8 o'clock to allow delivery of the head.

External cephalic version is still practised, but should not be performed prior to 37 weeks. Success rates vary: 48% (UK population); 93% (Black African women), resulting in reduced Caesarean section rates. It does have risks, those being premature labour, premature rupture of the membranes, abruption, cord entanglement, uterine rupture and fetal trauma. It should not be performed in patients with a previous scar on the uterus, twin pregnancies, oligohydramnios, fetal anomaly, hypertension or IUGR. Factors associated with failed ECV include difficulty in palpating the fetal head, the presenting part being engaged, and nulliparity. Although unproven, tocolysis may be of benefit for the tense uterus. If performed in rhesus negative patients then anti-D must be given and it should only be performed in a hospital where recourse to delivery is close at hand.

If contraindications are present then the use of Elkins' manoeuvre is advised, where the patient assumes the knee chest position for 15 minutes every 2 hours of waking time. It has been reported that approximately 90% of the babies underwent spontaneous version.

There is still much discussion about the desirability of vaginal breech delivery versus elective LSCS.

Wright in 1959 recommended routine Caesarean section for all breech presentations, because of the perceived increase in perinatal morbidity and mortality. In 1970 11.6% of breech presentations were delivered by LSCS; by 1993 this had increased to 63% in England, accounting for 15.5% of all Caesarean sections performed.

Caesarean section may decrease perinatal morbidity and mortality, but is associated with increased maternal mortality. Some studies have shown that the route of delivery for fetuses >1500 g does not affect perinatal mortality, or that the outcome may be poorer by abdominal delivery. There have only been a couple of randomized control trials that have compared the policy of planned Caesarean section with planned vaginal birth. An international multicentre study based in Canada is currently ongoing. The Cochrane database does not support routine elective Caesarean section, and recent evidence suggests that the long term outcome of infants delivered either by Caesarean section or planned vaginal delivery is associated with handicap or other health problems in 19.4%, regardless of mode of delivery.

The proportion of breech presentations diagnosed in labour varies between 9–33%. The undiagnosed breech is more likely to deliver vaginally, with no excess morbidity or mortality, compared to diagnosed breeches assessed for vaginal delivery. Thus there are no grounds for delivering all undiagnosed breeches by Caesarean section.

Further reading

Clinch J. Abnormal fetal presentations and positions. In: Turnbull Sir AC, Chamberlain GC. eds. *Obstetrics.* Edinburgh: Churchill Livingstone, 1991; **53:** 793–812.

Danielian PJ, Wang J, Hall MH. Long term outcome by method of delivery of fetuses in breech presentation at term: population based follow up. *British Medical Journal,* 1996; **312:** 1451–3.

Hannah M, Hannah W. Caesarean section or vaginal birth for breech presentation at term. *British Medical Journal,* 1996; **312:** 1433–4.

Lau TK, Keith WKLO, Wan D, Rogers MS. Predictors of successful ECV at term: a prospective study. *British Journal of Obstetrics and Gynaecology,* 1997; **104:** 798–802.

Nwosu EC, Walkinshaw S, Chia P, Manasse PR, Atlay RD. Undiagnosed breech. *British Journal of Obstetrics and Gynaecology,* 1993; **100:** 531–5.

Penn ZJ, Steer PJ, Grant A. A multicentre randomised control trial comparing elective and selective Caesarean section for the delivery of the preterm breech infant. *British Journal of Obstetrics and Gynaecology,* 1996; **103:** 684–9.

Thorpe-Beeston JG, Banfield PJ, Saunders NJ. Outcome of breech delivery at term. *British Medical Journal,* 1992; **305:** 746–7.

Related topics of interest

CAESAREAN SECTION

Caesarean section has become a much safer option for mother and baby. However, liberal use of Caesarean section, e.g. a rate >15% of all deliveries, has not been accompanied by a corresponding fall in perinatal mortality, and the procedure carries a significant morbidity whilst having implications for future pregnancies.

Lower segment Caesarean section

The introduction of the lower segment operation in the 1920s and 1930s was a major advance, causing less bleeding and a lower incidence of scar dehiscence. The widespread use of blood transfusion and introduction of antibiotics further improved the safety of the operation.

The uterus is usually approached via a Pfannenstiel incision and the lower segment incised transversely. Delivery of the baby and placenta is followed by closure of the uterus in two layers of a continuous absorbable suture, the first layer commonly being locked.

Indications

1. *Maternal.* Elective section is usually recommended if the patient has had two or more previous sections. Rarely, a patient is allowed to labour after two previous sections under carefully controlled situations.

The operation is recommended in patients with a history of cephalopelvic disproportion, especially if the baby is large and a narrow pelvis is demonstrated radiologically.

Placenta praevia of a grade to prevent vaginal delivery is likewise an absolute indication. Severe maternal illness may require delivery, by Caesarean section e.g. carcinoma of the cervix.

Emergency section may be required in fulminating pre-eclampsia, cephalopelvic disproportion or failed induction of labour.

2. *Fetal.* Elective section may be performed for multiple pregnancy or malpresentation.

Emergency section is performed for fetal distress and failed forceps.

Usually the decision to operate is taken after consideration of numerous factors, including past obstetric history, maternal age and fertility, maternal blood pressure, intercurrent illness, fetal maturity, fetal growth, evidence of fetal hypoxia from CTG, fetal blood sample and the presence of meconium. Decision-making should be the responsibility of senior staff.

Classical Caesarean section This procedure is now rarely performed mainly because of the higher rate of scar dehiscence in subsequent labour of about 9%. Subsequent delivery should always be by elective section.

The abdomen is entered via a lower midline or transverse incision. The uterus is incised vertically and may be repaired in three layers, particularly at the fundus, where the myometrium is thickest.

The classical approach gives more rapid access to the fetus, but the time difference is minimal and most surgeons are far more familiar with the lower-segment approach; consequently this procedure cannot be justified on the grounds of speed.

Indications 1. *Maternal.* The De Lee incision, which is a vertical incision over the lower part of the uterus, may be employed and is associated with a lower risk of subsequent scar dehiscence than a classical incision extending over the fundus.

2. *Fetal.* Malpresentation of the shoulder with a prolapsed arm and the fetal back directly beneath the lower segment.

Prematurity, such that the lower segment has not formed, a mass such as a fibroid obstructing the lower segment or adhesions over the lower segment.

Complications Operative complications are due to bleeding and bladder trauma. A lower segment incision may extend laterally to involve the uterine vessels. The ureters may be at risk in this situation.

Longitudinal incisions commonly cause significant haemorrhage. Rarely the lower segment incision needs to be converted to a 'J'- or a 'T'-shaped incision to facilitate a difficult delivery. Unrecognized bleeding may present in the immediate post-operative period; infection in the uterus, pelvis or wound presents in the first week and is related to prolonged rupture of membranes.

The scar may dehisce in subsequent labour; the prevalence is less than 0.5% after a lower segment operation but higher after classical section.

Further reading

Beazley JM. Caesarean section. In: Turnbull Sir AC, Chamberlain GC, eds. *Obstetrics.* Edinburgh: Churchill Livingstone, 1989: 857–65.

Related topics of interest

Cephalopelvic disproportion (p. 188)
Perioperative complications in obstetrics and gynaecology (p. 100)
Puerperal sepsis (p. 300)
Report on Confidential Enquiries into Maternal Deaths in the United Kingdom 1991–1993 (p. 309)

CANCER IN PREGNANCY

Cancer complicates about 1 in 1000 pregnancies. Management is complex and should be individualized, taking into account the site and stage of the disease, the gestation and the general health of both mother and fetus. The prospective parents should be kept fully informed and included at all stages in management discussion. Treatment is formulated using a multidisciplinary approach, including obstetrician, surgical and medical oncologists and radiotherapists where applicable. Ideally the patient should be referred to a centre with the necessary expertise.

Principles of management

The prognosis of cancer is related to the stage of the disease. Cure rates are higher in early-stage disease, and treatment should not be deferred for any significant length of time to allow fetal maturity to occur.

In general, early pregnancies should be terminated to allow treatment of the cancer to commence. In later pregnancy treatment may be deferred for a week or two to allow the fetus to mature. The exact timing of intervention is a matter decided after discussion between all clinicians involved, taking into account the parents' wishes.

Treatment of the cancer is as for the non-pregnant patient; the fetus is adversely affected by cytotoxic chemotherapy, especially in the first trimester, and radiotherapy to the abdomen and pelvis.

There is a risk of abortion with general anaesthesia, which will increase with the duration of the surgical procedure and the site of surgery if in anatomical relation to the gravid uterus.

Pelvic cancer and pregnancy

The quoted prevalence of carcinoma of the cervix in pregnancy is 1–13 in 10 000. Vaginal delivery is contraindicated because of the increased risk of dissemination of malignant cells via the local lymphatics and blood vessels.

The prognosis is not altered by pregnancy, stage for stage. Termination of early pregnancy is followed by radical surgery or radiotherapy as appropriate. In later pregnancy a Caesarean Wertheim radical hysterectomy or a standard Caesarean section may be performed, followed by radiotherapy, if appropriate.

A recent report described the use of neo-adjuvent cisplatinum in cervical cancer administered at 22, 25 and 28 weeks gestation with no adverse effect on the fetus.

Forty cases of cancer of the vulva during pregnancy have been reported in the literature. Radical vulvectomy and bilateral groin node dissection may be performed in the first half of pregnancy. Vaginal delivery may be allowed if the lesion is remote from the introitus; similarly, vaginal delivery can be allowed after radical vulval surgery, with appropriate care of the perineum at delivery.

Carcinoma of the ovary in pregnancy is rare. Differentiation from a physiological cyst is based on ultrasonic features such as an enlarging cyst with septae and solid areas. Surgical exploration is performed in doubtful cases. Treatment is as for the non-pregnant and prognosis is unaltered stage for stage.

Carcinoma of the vagina and corpus uteri is extremely rare in pregnancy.

Other primary pelvic malignancies, e.g. of the rectum and bladder, are rare. The fetus is unlikely to be unaffected by radical pelvic surgery, but if mature Caesarean section may be performed as a preliminary procedure.

Extrapelvic cancer and pregnancy

The incidence of breast cancer in pregnancy increases with maternal age. The general prognosis is worse than normal with a 5-year survival of about 25% because of the delay in diagnosis due to physiological enlargement of the breast and because there is early metastasis as a result of the increased blood supply to the breast and a preponderance of unfavourable histological types.

Breast surgery and local radiotherapy may be performed if adequate precautions to protect the fetus are observed. However, cytotoxic chemotherapy warrants termination.

If there is no evidence of recurrence then pregnancy may be allowed with no adverse effect after successful treatment of breast cancer.

Leukaemias and lymphomas (especially Hodgkin's disease) are relatively common in women of child-bearing years. Cytotoxic chemotherapy is the mainstay of treatment and may be administered from the second trimester with careful selection of cytotoxic agents to minimize fetal risk. Fertility is often preserved and subsequent pregnancy is safe after a reasonable interval of about 2 years.

Melanoma appears to be adversely affected by pregnancy and treatment should be promptly instituted.

Hormone-dependent thyroid cancers are stimulated by the TSH effect of the gonadotrophins and prompt termination should be recommended.

Cancer and the fetus
Metastases to the fetus and placenta are extremely rare, with 53 documented cases. The cancer likely to metastasize to this site is malignant melanoma.

Further reading

Ciacalone PL *et al.* Cisplatinum neoadjuvant chemotherapy in a pregnant woman with invasive carcinoma of the uterine cervix. *British Journal of Obstetrics and Gynaecology,* 1996; **103:** 932–4.

Shepherd JH. Cancer complicating pregnancy. In: Shepherd JH, Monaghan JM, eds. *Clinical Gynaecological Oncology*, 2nd edn. Oxford: Blackwell Scientific Publications, 1990; 351–70.

Related topics of interest

Abortion, spontaneous/recurrent (p. 7)
Cancer of the cervix (p. 16)
Gestational trophoblastic disease (p. 44)
Ovarian tumours: epithelial (p. 87)
Ovarian tumours: non-epithelial (p. 90)
Vulva (p. 151)

CARDIAC DISEASE IN PREGNANCY

Cardiac disease in pregnancy is significant, accounting for 41 deaths in the latest Triennial Confidential Enquiries into Maternal Deaths. Congenital heart disease accounted for 21% of the deaths. Substandard care was present in 27% of these deaths. A notable feature was that nine of the deaths were due to a ruptured thoracic aortic aneurysm. By way of comparison the prevalence of cardiac disease in the Western world is of the order of 1%.

Management and treatment Whenever there is a known diagnosis it is helpful if advice is sought from a cardiologist prior to achieving a pregnancy, and thereafter the pregnant cardiac patient should be managed by a cardiologist and an obstetrician with an interest, i.e. in a high-risk pregnancy unit. Historically the cardinal symptom is dyspnoea, but because most pregnant women experience this it can be difficult to grade. Syncopal attacks and palpitations secondary to arrhythmias may occur, whereas chest pain is uncommon.

Examination findings will reveal the normal hyperdynamics of pregnancy, murmurs of all varieties dependent upon the underlying pathology, with or without signs of cardiac failure, cyanosis and endocarditis. Chest radiology will show the normal cardiomegaly, increased pulmonary vascularity, with or without the pathology, whilst electocardiographic changes in normal pregnancy include T wave inversion in III, S-T segment changes and Q waves. The ECG is probably best at detecting the arrhythmias of pregnancy. Echocardiography is very useful.

Once diagnosed one must ascertain the severity of a cardiac lesion in pregnancy. Continuation with the pregnancy as a risk to a woman's life must be evaluated. Eisenmenger's syndrome (30% mortality if the pregnancy continues versus 7% mortality for termination) and primary pulmonary hypertension are absolute contraindications to continuation and the pregnancy should be terminated. Cardiac surgery for other lesions is decided upon the merits of the cardiac lesion. Regular antenatal review and assessment is necessary, with strict attention paid to maternal and fetal health.

Heart failure, if and when it occurs, is treated in the usual way with digoxin. Digoxin crosses the placental barrier and is excreted in breast milk, but provided the mother remains within therapeutic levels there is no evidence of digoxin toxicity to the fetus or neonate. Diuretics are used where necessary, but there is a risk of hypokalaemia. Morphine and/or aminophylline are used for pulmonary oedema. Rarely, mechanical ventilation is necessary, but, if so, cardiac surgery should be offered if the lesion is surgically correctable.

Labour

Induction of labour should be evaluated on merit. Most cardiac patients in pregnancy will tolerate epidural anaesthesia. The second stage should not exceed the normal parameters, but elective forceps deliveries are not always necessary. Syntocinon is the drug of choice in the third stage (to avoid the 500 ml bolus of blood 'squeezed' into the maternal systemic circulation from the use of ergometrine), but in a post-partum haemorrhage use of ergometrine is essential. The addition of IV frusemide may conteract the tendency to pulmonary oedema in such cases. Endocarditis is a risk in such cases, and this has been specifically targeted by the Confidential Enquiries into Maternal Deaths. Ampicillin, 500 mg IM at 8-hourly intervals for three doses and gentamicin 80 mg IM at 8-hourly intervals for three doses (check renal function and monitor levels) are the drugs of choice, with vancomycin, 500 mg IV in two doses at 12-hour intervals being reserved for the penicillin-sensitive patient.

Heart valves

The pregnant patient with an artificial heart valve deserves special mention, her main problem being one of anticoagulation. Fetal and maternal morbidity and mortality are significantly higher in this group of patients. Despite the associated embryopathy, warfarin is the drug of choice in such patients.

Other conditions

- Myocardial infarction: this is rare (frequency 1:10 000), with a 40% mortality. PET is an association.
- Cardiomyopathy: may be pregnancy specific.
- Coarctation of the aorta and Marfan's: maternal risk of dissection. Delivery by section is probably best if there is aortic disease.

- Heart block: this is generally no problem, but pacing may be necessary.

Further reading

De Swiet M. Cardiovascular problems in pregnancy. In: Turnbull Sir AC, Chamberlain GC, eds. *Obstetrics*. Edinburgh: Churchill Livingstone, 1989; 543–55.

Related topics of interest

Physiology of pregnancy (p. 260)
Pre-eclampsia, eclampsia and phaeochromocytoma (p. 270)

CEPHALOPELVIC DISPROPORTION

Defined as the failure of the head to pass through the pelvis safely because the pelvis is too small and/or the head too large.

The more serious consequences of cephalopelvic disproportion are uterine rupture, vesicovaginal fistula, maternal and fetal death and birth injury.

The pelvis which bounds the birth canal has an important weight bearing function. The formation and consolidation of the bone depends on adequate amounts of calcium, vitamin D and phosphorous. Therefore rickets and osteomalacia would effect this bone formation and therefore can result in a small pelvis; this is especially relevant in developing countries. The pattern of pelvic contraction in a community reflects the diet of the females. This is especially noted in the immigrant Asian patient in the UK.

Causes
    (a) Pelvic shape.
    (b) Size of the baby.
    (c) Space occupying lesions, e.g. ovarian cyst.

Pelvic shape
The relationship between stature and size of pelvis is well known. Women in their first pregnancies who are <155 cm (5'1") and who have a shoe size <3 need to be watched. In these cases antenatal pelvic assessment may be indicated.

In Afro-Caribbean patients the fetal head is often high because of the high angle of inclination of their pelvis.

However, non-engagement of the head at the onset of labour is important and CPD should be suspected if engagement does not occur after 39 weeks.

Vaginal examination can help. One must assess the subpubic angle, the anteroposterior diameter to the sacrum and both the interspinous and intertuberous diameters.

Expectant management of suspected CPD in a primigravida is a trial of labour.

If possible, prior to labour X-ray pelvimetry is useful, although CT scan or an MRI scan are now better, as they give a three dimensional picture.

Size of baby
This is particularly important in the small woman and also in the diabetic patient where macrosomia can occur. It is important to remember that babies can increase in size, so that if a woman has had a normal vaginal delivery with her first baby it *does not* mean

that she will have a vaginal delivery with the second baby.

Space occupying lesion

The most important of these are an ovarian cyst or a cervical fibroid.

Discussion

CPD in labour in a primigravid patient can be suspected if the following occurs:

- Head remains three fifths to four fifths palpable per abdomen.
- Prolonged latent phase.
- Active phase dilatation is retarded (often stops 7–9 cm).
- Poor application of the cervix to the head.
- Excessive head moulding with caput.
- Impaction of the head may prevent anterior rotation.
- Fetal heart rate abnormalities on the CTG.

If cephalopelvic disproportion is suspected, then recourse to Caesarean section is essential for safety of both mother and baby. If a woman has not delivered within 12 hours of regular contractions, then the situation must be reassessed.

Vaginal delivery should not be attempted in questionable cases if fetal distress is present. If a trial of vaginal delivery is attempted then it should be performed in a theatre that is equipped to perform a LSCS straight away.

CPD in parous women is a much more dangerous problem as it is often unsuspected. Diagnosis of mechanical difficulty rests on other features in labour, namely, delay in descent of the head, exaggerated moulding and sometimes unremitting uterine activity.

The classical signs of impending spontaneous rupture of an unscarred uterus such as frequent violent uterine contractions and an exaggerated retraction ring (Bandl's ring) do not usually appear prior to rupture.

Further reading

Anon. Rickets in Asian immigrants. (Editorial). *British Medical Journal*, 1979; **1:** 1744.

Myerscough P. Cephalopelvic disproportion. In: Turnbull Sir AC, Chamberlain GC, eds. *Obstetrics*. Edinburgh: Churchill Livingstone, 1991; **54:** 813–21.

Related topics of interest

Anatomy of the female pelvis, the fetal skull and the fetal circulation (p. 166)
Breech (p. 175)
Caesarean section (p. 179)

COAGULATION AND PREGNANCY

Physiology

Blood clotting is determined by three factors described originally by Virchow: blood flow, integrity of blood vessel walls and coagulability of the blood. The last-mentioned depends on platelet function, the extrinsic and intrinsic clotting cascade and the fibrinolytic system.

Pregnancy alters the flow of blood. The vessels are generally dilated and blood pressure is lower, tending to cause stasis of flow. Vessel walls and platelet count are not significantly influenced by pregnancy alone, although there is probably an increased turnover of platelets.

The coagulation system is altered in favour of clot formation, designed to limit blood loss at parturition. Significant increases in the concentration of clotting factors II, VII, VIII and X occur, especially in the placenta, and there is fibrin deposition (replacing elastic and muscle tissue within the placental vessels, thereby increasing blood flow). Fibrinolytic activity is inhibited, again resulting in clot formation, especially in the placenta, where no detectable plasminogen activator is found.

Thromboembolism

Pregnancy increases the risk of thromboembolism sixfold, affecting between 0.3 and 1.2% of all pregnancies. Factors are related to Virchow's triad as described above, with increased stasis in the veins of the lower limbs due to pressure of the gravid uterus. Venous stasis is increased with prolonged bed rest.

Major risk factors

- Hereditary thrombophilia, e.g. antithrombin III deficiency.
- Anti-phospholipid syndrome. Positive anticardiolipin antibodies or lupus anticoagulant.
- Method of delivery: LSCS carries a 10-fold increased risk compared with vaginal delivery.

Associated risk factors

- Age >35 years.
- Increasing parity (4 or more).

- Obesity >76 kg.
- Previous history of DVT or PE.
- Prolonged recumbency.
- Family history of pulmonary embolism.
- Hypertension.
- Infection.
- Chronic illness.
- Gross varicose veins.

Deep venous thrombosis presents with a hot, painful and red swelling of the affected leg. Diagnosis may be confirmed by Doppler ultrasound, although venography may be performed if the abdomen is protected. Treatment is commenced on clinical grounds and the diagnosis confirmed later.

Pulmonary embolus, if massive, presents with acute collapse. Chest pain, dyspnoea and haemoptysis may suggest the diagnosis, which is confirmed by ventilation-perfusion isotope scan. This remains a major cause of maternal mortality with 35 reported deaths in the most recent Confidential Enquiry into Maternal Deaths. Treatment is with intravenous heparin, to prevent further clot formation and minimize the risk of embolization. For maintenance therapy and prophylaxis the choice is between warfarin and subcutaneous heparin.

Warfarin is given orally. The drug crosses the placenta and is associated with abortion, congenital abnormality and fetal intracerebral bleeding. Women on long-term warfarin have a fetal mortality rate of 15%. Warfarin embryopathy is related to drug administration at around 6–9 weeks' gestation and comprises; saddle nose, nasal and mid-face hypoplasia, frontal bossing, short stature, calcification of thyroid cartilage, cardiac lesions, low-set ears, mental retardation and blindness.

The drug should not be given in late pregnancy as it is difficult to reverse its anticoagulant effect.

Heparin does not cross the placenta, is not teratogenic and is easily reversed with protamine sulphate. It has to be administered by injection, which may cause bruising. There may be an associated thrombocytopaenia.

There have been reports of osteopaenia causing back pain and vertebral collapse associated with long-term use.

Low molecular weight heparins are administered once daily and are less likely to cause osteopaenia.

Recent guidelines suggest low molecular weight heparin as the agent of choice in antenatal prophylaxis.

Disseminated intravascular coagulation

This is always a secondary phenomenon with stimulation of the clotting system to produce intravascular coagulation with consequent consumption of clotting factors and platelets leading to haemorrhage. Many pregnancy-related factors may trigger DIC, including pre-eclampsia, abruptio placentae, uterine infection, large fetomaternal transfusion, retained dead fetus or products of conception, hydatidiform mole and amniotic fluid embolism.

Management depends on prompt recognition of the disorder with immediate and adequate replacement therapy with blood, fresh-frozen plasma, platelets and calcium. Clotting factors are used in extreme cases. Accurate fluid balance is essential and transfusion requirements are dictated by the results of frequent estimation of haematological indices.

Intravenous heparin may be administered in an attempt to break the cycle of clot formation and breakdown when the circulatory system is intact.

Further reading

De Swiet M. Thromboembolism. In: De Swiet M, ed. *Medical Disorders in Obstetric Practice*, 2nd edn. Oxford: Blackwell Scientific Publications, 1989; 166–97.

Letsky EA. Coagulation defects. In: De Swiet M, ed. *Medical Disorders in Obstetric Practice*, 2nd edn. Oxford: Blackwell Scientific Publications, 1989; 104–65.

Report of the RCOG Working Party on Prophylaxis Against Thromboembolism in Gynaecology and Obstetrics. London: RCOG Publication, 1995.

Related topics of interest

Antepartum haemorrhage (p. 169)

Pre-eclampsia, eclampsia and phaeochromocytoma (p. 270)

Report on Confidential Enquiries into Maternal Deaths in the United Kingdom 1991–1993 (p. 309)

CONFIDENTIAL ENQUIRY INTO STILLBIRTHS AND DEATHS IN INFANCY (CESDI)

The fourth annual report of CESDI was released in April, 1997. It is the first report prepared under the auspices of the Maternal and Child Health Research consortium, a body convened and run specifically for the Enquiry with representatives from the Royal College of Obstetricians and Gynaecologists, the Royal College of Midwives, the Royal College of Paediatrics and Child Health and the Royal College of Pathologists. CESDI was established in 1992 to collect information on late fetal losses, stillbirths and deaths in infancy, with a view to identifying ways in which these deaths might be prevented.

In 1994 and 1995, 19 348 deaths between 20 weeks of pregnancy and one year of age were reported to CESDI, covering England, Wales and Northern Ireland. In the same period there were 1 359 368 live births. It appears that intrapartum mortality rates have stayed static for a number of years. Of the total number of deaths reported to CESDI, 1266 (6.5%) were subjected to a confidential enquiry. Of these enquired cases, there were 873 deaths from intrapartum-related events (1 in 1561 births) and these deaths created 3265 separate comments. These deaths are the main focus of this report.

Over 78% of these intrapartum-related deaths were criticized for suboptimal care, because alternative management 'might' (25%) or 'would reasonably be expected to' (52%) have made a difference to outcome. The dominant problem in antepartum care was the management of risk factors, including identification and consequent treatment plans. The dominant problem in intrapartum care was the assessment of fetal condition by heart rate monitoring and blood sampling.

Of the 1266 cases subjected to confidential enquiry, 38% had no form of autopsy. The placenta was sent for histological examination in less than 50% of cases. Even where an autopsy was performed, one-fifth of cases did not have histological reports.

A number of recommendations and future developments came out of this report covering training, assessment and supervision of midwives and obstetricians, the role of Royal Colleges, pathology and autopsy, the quality of maternity records, guidelines covering all aspects of fetal assessment before and during labour (ideally at national level), communication between professionals and parents, standardizing definitions and the future role of CESDI.

As for CEMD and NCEPOD, this report is mandatory reading for all obstetricians, midwives and paediatricians and pathologists.

Further reading

CESDI Confidential Enquiry into Stillbirths and Deaths in Infancy. 4th Annual Report. 1 January–31 December, 1995. Maternal and Child Health Research Consortium, April, 1997.

Related topics of interest

Report on Confidential Enquiries into Maternal Deaths in the United Kingdom, 1991–1993 (p. 309)

DIABETES AND PREGNANCY

Diabetes is a clinical syndrome characterized by hyperglycaemia owing to a deficiency or diminished effectiveness of insulin. Pregnancy is a diabetogenic condition owing to the anti-insulin effects of pregnancy-related hormones such as human placental lactogen and cortisol. The insulin-resistant state of pregnancy is most marked in the third trimester. Undiagnosed or poorly treated diabetes in pregnancy has significant implications for a woman's antenatal, intrapartum and post-natal progress. Maternal glucose crosses over the placenta into the fetal circulation by facilitated diffusion and hence the fetal blood glucose closely mirrors that of the mother. Thus the fetus may be adversely affected if the maternal condition is ignored.

Diagnosis

A recent report by The Pregnancy and Neonatal Care Group recommended the following criteria for screening and diagnosis of diabetes in pregnancy:

1. Urine should be tested for glycosuria at every antenatal visit.
2. Timed random laboratory blood glucose measurements should be made:

- whenever glycosuria (1+ or more) is detected.
- at the booking visit and at 28 weeks gestation.
- A 75 g oral glucose tolerance test (GTT) should be done if the timed random blood glucose concentrations are:
  (a) >6 mmol/l in the fasting state of 2 hours after food, or
  (b) >7 mmol/l within 2 hours of food.

If the timed random blood glucose measurement exceeds 11 mmol/l, then the GTT should be omitted and pre- and postprandial blood glucose measurements on an appropriate diet should be performed to assess the need for insulin.

Interpreting a 75 g oral GTT in pregnancy

	Plasma glucose	
	Fasting (mmol/l)	2 hours (mmol/l)
Diabetes	>8	>11
Gestational impaired glucose tolerance	6–8	9–11
Normal	<6	<9

Indications for GTT

- Previous diabetes, stillbirth, neonatal death, congenital anomaly or big baby > 4.5 kg.
- Obesity > 20% above ideal body weight.
- Polyhydramnios.
- Development of fetal macrosomia.
- Glycosuria on more than two occasions.
- Positive family history.

A glycosylated haemoglobin assay, HbA_{1C}, may also be used to aid diagnosis, prospectively or retrospectively, as glycosylation may be significantly raised in diabetes (normal population glycosylation, 4%; diabetic population, >10%).

Treatment

Insulin is the drug of choice in a diabetic pregnancy. Oral hypoglycaemics are not recommended. Most regimens use a mixture of short-acting and long-acting insulins, with the proportions of each initially being determined by trial and error in the newly diagnosed diabetic. Self-monitoring is vital, and some clinics now draw upon the technology of glucometers with a capacity to store the preceding 2 weeks' results, which can then be printed out in the clinic.

Classification

The severity of diabetes in pregnancy may be classified along the lines of King's College Hospital criteria, and this is useful as the more severe the classification then the more likely is the potential for maternal and fetal problems:

Group 1: diabetes diagnosed during the pregnancy (i.e. gestational diabetes, which by definition reverts to a non-diabetic state post-partum).

Group 2: established diabetes with less than six microaneurysms on ophthalmoscopy.

Group 3: established diabetes with more than six microaneurysms on ophthalmoscopy or proliferative retinopathy and/or nephropathy.

Management

The ideal medical management of a diabetic pregnancy is in a clinic shared by an obstetrician and diabetic physician. Ideally there should be a diabetes specialist midwife, who will be available to the diabetic in labour. Referral to a medical ophthalmologist is important if the woman has not been seen in the past year, or if she develops visual symptoms or signs. Ultrasound scanning, especially anomaly and fetal size scanning, should be routine. A dietitian is essential.

Complications

The pregnant diabetic patient is particularly prone to three complications, namely pre-eclampsia with a prevalence of 14.4%, polyhydramnios with a prevalence of 25%, and pre-term labour with a prevalence of around 17%. Fetuses of diabetic mothers have delayed lung maturation due to hyperglycaemia inhibiting surfactant production, and they may exhibit respiratory distress syndrome (RDS) up to 37 weeks' gestation, especially if diabetic control has been suboptimal. Tocolysis with beta-sympathomimetics and acceleration of fetal lung maturity with corticosteroids are indicated, as for the non-diabetic pre-term labour, in conjunction with normoglycaemia and prevention of hypokalaemia.

Delivery

Delivery of the pregnant diabetic should be planned as an induction of labour at 38–40 weeks' gestation if all is well. Every effort should be made to ensure that the labour progresses uneventfully with avoidance of prolonged or difficult labours. In general, the rule of elective Caesarean section in a diabetic pregnancy with a complication, e.g. severe pre-eclampsia or a breech presentation, should be observed. Even centres of excellence will have a Caesarean section rate of at least 30% in pregnant diabetics. The labouring diabetic patient will have her fetus continuously monitored with a cardiotocograph, hourly blood glucose assessments, an insulin infusion into one arm and a 10% dextrose infusion to the other. The aim is for a blood glucose of 4–6 mmol/l, with constant insulin infusion adjustments accordingly. One should augment labour 'sooner rather than later', and epidural anaesthesia is not contraindicated.

Post-partum

The post-partum diabetic mother should be encouraged to breast feed (but warned of the possibility of hypoglycaemia, which can be sudden during breast feeding), and contraception should be discussed prior to leaving hospital. The low-dose triphasic pill or the progesterone-only pill is recommended if she chooses oral contraception, although there is an increased risk of thromboembolism. Obesity and smoking should be strongly resisted in such women. The IUCD, sheath, or diaphragm will appeal to some, and sterilization should be offered to those who have completed their family.

The fetus and neonate   The fetus of a diabetic mother is at risk of early spontaneous abortion, growth retardation or macrosomia, asphyxia (33% will require intubation at delivery), hypoglycaemia, hypocalcaemia, hypomagnesaemia, RDS, polycythaemia, jaundice and birth trauma and has a 7% chance of major congenital anomalies. They have a 10-fold greater chance of developing diabetes in later life than infants of non-diabetic mothers (1% versus 0.1%). CNS development is generally normal, although neurological abnormality is possible if there has been prolonged neonatal hypoglycaemia. The caudal regression syndrome is pathognomonic of a diabetic pregnancy with a prevalence of 1:1000 diabetic pregnancies.

Further reading

Brudenell M. Diabetic pregnancy. In: Turnbull Sir AC, Chamberlain GC, eds. *Obstetrics.* Edinburgh: Churchill Livingstone, 1989; 585–603.
Jardine Brown, C *et al.* Report of the Pregnancy and Neonatal Care Group. *Diabetic Medicine,* 1996; **13:** S43–S53.

Related topics of interest

Immunology of pregnancy (p. 225)
Pre-eclampsia, eclampsia and phaeochromocytoma (p. 270)

DIAGNOSIS OF PREGNANCY

History (symptoms)

1. Amenorrhoea. The first missed period occurs at approximately 14 days post fertilization; implantation bleeding may mask this symptom.

2. Nausea and vomiting. This is usually noticed after amenorrhoea, a common symptom but often not confined to mornings.

3. Breast symptoms. The earliest is of tingling in the breasts, most frequently noticed by primigravida. Later discomfort and nipple discoloration may occur. Nipple discharge may occasionally occur but is commoner in late pregnancy.

4. Urinary symptoms. Usually frequency, this occurs at 8–10 weeks' gestation.

Examination (signs)

1. Breasts. The breasts may be soft and globular. An easier sign to detect is increased nipple pigmentation and the presence of Montgomery's tubercles. These signs appear from about 8 weeks' gestation. Later the veins just beneath the skin of the breast become prominent, especially around the nipple.

2. Uterus. The uterus enlarges and becomes soft and globular and likewise the cervix softens. These signs may be detectable from 6 weeks' gestation.

Examination with a speculum, looking for a blue discoloration of the cervix and bimanual examination to elicit Hegar's sign are unnecessarily traumatic and should not be performed.

3. Abdomen. The enlarged uterus is palpable abdominally by 12–13 weeks. Pregnancy should be excluded in any woman of reproductive years presenting with an abdominal mass arising from the pelvis.

Investigation

The diagnosis of pregnancy has become much more sophisticated with the advent of enzyme-linked immunosorbent assay. This allows identification of the beta subunit of hCG, which is specific at low concentrations of 25–50 IU per litre. These concentrations occur at about 10 days post fertilization, i.e. before the missed period. This test is available commercially and has eliminated the false positives obtained with less specific tests due to cross- reaction with other (alpha) subunits present on LH, FSH and TSH.

Ultrasound may detect a gestation sac by 5–6 weeks' gestation, its main role is to diagnose a viable pregnancy (by visualization of a beating fetal heart) at 7–8 weeks' gestation. Ultrasound diagnosis is at an earlier stage (i.e. 5 weeks) when a transvaginal probe is ulitized.

A portable Doppler ultrasound probe may detect an audible fetal heart at 12 weeks' gestation and is a valuable adjunct in the booking clinic, as well as reassuring anxious prospective parents.

Further reading

Chamberlain GC. Diagnosis of pregnancy. In: Turnbull Sir AC, Chamberlain GC. eds. *Obstetrics*. Edinburgh: Churchill Livingstone, 1989; 219–23.

Related topics of interest

Physiology of pregnancy (p. 260)
Prenatal diagnosis (p. 281)

DRUGS IN PREGNANCY: ANTIBIOTICS, ANALGESICS AND ANTICONVULSANTS

The general advice given to patients is to avoid all drugs in the first trimester, unless treatment is absolutely necessary. Teratogenic effects are manifest mainly in early pregnancy before organogenesis is complete. The incidence of teratogenic effects will vary depending on the offending drug, with cytotoxic agents such as methotrexate being invariably harmful but others such as the anticonvulsants causing teratogenic effects in only a proportion of affected pregnancies.

The advice given to patients should be that treatment should not be withheld when it is necessary, e.g. in asthmatic attacks, but the mother should be informed of any potential risk to her and the fetus.

Antibiotics

The choice of antibiotic is governed by the site of infection, whether the fetus is alive *in utero* and the results of bacteriological investigation.

Tetracyclines are contraindicated as they stain fetal teeth, chloramphenicol causes the 'grey baby' syndrome, sulphonamides cause neonatal haemolysis and trimethoprim is a folate antagonist.

The urinary tract is the commonest site of infection in pregnancy, and amoxycillin or co-amoxiclav is usually effective. Erythromycin may be given to penicillin-sensitive patients and trimethoprim is safe in the mid-trimester (folic acid supplements may be given).

Respiratory infections are frequently of viral aetiology. If antibiotics are indicated then amoxycillin or erythromycin is usually given.

Antibiotic prophylaxis is indicated for Caesarean section and a single dose of intravenous co-amoxiclav is commonly given at operation.

Antibiotic prophylaxis may be indicated in premature rupture of the membranes, especially if beta-haemolytic streptococci are cultured from the vagina. Benzylpenicillin is commonly used for this purpose, although a broader spectrum antibiotic may be preferred.

For pelvic or intra-abdominal infection efficacy against anaerobic bacteria is necessary and metronidazole should be added to a broad-spectrum agent such as cefuroxime.

Information is limited as to the safety of more recently developed antibiotics, such as ciprofloxacin, and their use should be confined to life-threatening infections until their safety in pregnancy is established.

Analgesics

The safety of paracetamol in pregnancy is well established, and this is the analgesic agent of choice for mild pain.

Non-steroidal anti-inflammatory agents cause premature closure of the fetal ductus arteriosus and may predispose to haemorrhage, especially at delivery. Aspirin in low dose has a significant inhibitory effect on platelet function. It is given in combination with heparin in women with antiphospholipid syndrome.

Opiate analgesics are commonly prescribed for severe pain in pregnancy, especially during labour, when pethidine is the most popular drug. It has a relatively short duration of action and is less likely to cause depression of neonatal respiratory effort than other opiates, although this will depend on the time interval between administration and delivery. If there is significant inhibition of neonatal respiration then the opiate antagonist naloxone may be given. Another opiate effect is gastric stasis, which predisposes to aspiration pneumonitis in the mother. Papaveretum is no longer administered to pregnant women as it contains noscapine, which may be teratogenic.

Anticonvulsants

The first report of congenital abnormalities in infants born to mothers who had taken anticonvulsants in pregnancy was in 1968. Since then numerous reports have linked anticonvulsants with a variety of malformations. Cleft lip and palate, cardiac and facial anomalies and neural tube defects have all been reported. These last have a particular association with sodium valproate, although the folate antagonist property of anticonvulsants may theoretically predispose to neural tube defects.

In general terms the dose of anticonvulsants given to a pregnant woman should be kept to the minimum necessary to avoid convulsions. The teratogenic potential should be explained, but the risk of seizures is such that drug therapy should be maintained. Folic acid supplements (4 mg daily) should also be prescribed.

Conclusions   Essential drug treatment should not be withheld from pregnant women. They should be informed of the risks of teratogenic and other side-effects. If possible, a drug with a superior safety record should be prescribed. In general, it is best to avoid non-essential medication, especially in the first trimester.

Further reading

Hopkins A. Neurological disorders. In: De Swiet M, ed. *Medical Disorders in Obstetric Practice*, 2nd edn. Oxford: Blackwell Scientific Publications, 1989; 731–74.

Kelleher CJ, Cardozo LA, Antimicrobials in pregnancy. In: Studd J, ed. *Progress in Obstetrics and Gynaecology,* Vol. 10. Edinburgh: Churchill Livingstone, 1993: 111–33.

Related topics of interest

Analgesia/anaesthesia in labour (p. 163)
Epilepsy and pregnancy (p. 208)
Infection in pregnancy (p. 232)
Preterm rupture of the membranes (PROM) (p. 293)

EMBRYOLOGY

Embryology must cover both the female genital tract and the urinary system. Each overlaps the other but for simplicity they will be described separately.

Urinary system

The majority arises from the intermediate cell mass (mesoderm). Two nephrogenic ridges each side of the midline arise and go from the cervical region down to the caudal end of the fetus. Three sets of structures appear successively, the pronephros which regresses totally, the mesonephros which will give rise to the glomerular capsule and collecting ducts which initially empty into the longitudinal collecting duct called the mesonephric or Wolffian duct.

The mesonephros degenerates in a craniocaudal direction and has disappeared by the third month. Two vestigial structures will remain in the adult female, non-functioning tubules of the epoophoron, which lie in the broad ligament and the paroophoron, which lies medial to the ovary.

The metanephros develops from two sources, firstly the ureteric bud from the mesonephric duct and secondly the metanephrogenic cap from the intermediate cell mass of the lower lumbar and sacral regions.

The ureteric bud outgrowth of the mesonephric duct near where the latter opens into the anterior part of the cloaca grows into the metonephrogenic cap, and will form the ureter. The mesodermal cells of the metanephrogenic cap the glomerular capsules, the proximal and distal convoluted tubules and the loops of Henlé. Each division of the ureteric bud will have its own cap of mesoderm.

The metanephros is at first a pelvic organ receiving its blood supply from the middle sacral artery. It will ascend up the posterior abdominal wall eventually coming to lie opposite the second lumbar vertebrae.

The bladder develops from the anterior portion of the cloaca which has been previously separated into anterior and posterior parts by the urorectal septum.

The mesonephric ducts enter into the anterior part of the cloaca. The caudal parts of the mesonephric ducts become absorbed into the lower part of the bladder so that the ureters and ducts have individual openings. Because of differential growth, the ureters open through the lateral angles of the bladder and the mesonephric ducts open close together in what will be the future urethra. This part of the bladder wall marked by the four openings is called the trigone. The early stage lining over the trigone is mesodermal, later to be replaced by epithelium of entodermal origin.

The primitive bladder is divided into an upper dilated portion, the bladder (with the allantois from its apex to the umbilicus thus forming the adult urachus), and the lower narrow portion, the urethra.

The mesonephric duct as described gives rise to the ureteric bud, but otherwise largely disappears. Small remnants persist as the duct of the epoophoron and the duct of the paroophoron, as described earlier. The caudal end may persist and extend from the epoophoron to the hymen as Gartner's duct.

The female urethra is derived from the mesonephric ducts forming the upper two-thirds and the lower end from the urogenital sinus.

Female genital tract

Primordial sex cells are first seen in the wall of the yolk sac close to the allantois. These cells will migrate to lie on the medial side of the mesonephros; they grow down into the mesenchyme and are called sex cords. They will form a ridge called the genital ridge. At this stage development is the same for male and female.

The ovary develops from the primordial sex cells that form oogonia; these will later form the primary oocytes that will be surrounded by a single layer of cells called granulosa cells, thus forming the primordial follicle. The surrounding mesenchyme will form the ovarian stroma.

Paramesonephric ducts develop on the lateral side of the mesonephric ducts as invagination of coelomic epithelium into the underlying mesenchyme. The cranial end will retain its ostium around which will develop the fimbriae. The caudal end will grow down laterally to the mesonephric duct and on reaching the pelvis it will cross ventrally to reach its medial side and join its opposite number. The combined caudal ends will reach the posterior wall of the urogenital sinus.

As the paramesonephric ducts descend through the pelvis anterior to the developing rectum and posterior to the primitive bladder, they pull toward the midline a transverse fold of coelomic epithelium and underlying mesenchyme on each side, which will result in the adult broad ligament.

The paramesonephric ducts will form the Fallopian tubes, the uterine body and cervix.

The vagina will be formed from the urogenital sinus. Two sinovaginal bulbs develop from the urogenital sinus at the site where the paramesonephric ducts enter. The cells of the sinovaginal bulbs proliferate to form the vaginal plate, which plate extends completely around the cervix formed by the fused paramesonephric ducts.

The plate will thicken and elongate and then canalize. The hymen develops from the distal part of the vaginal plate and the wall of the urogenital sinus.

Further reading

Beck F, Moffat DB, Lloyd JB. *Human Embryology and Genetics*. Blackwell Scientific Publications,1973; 241–60.

Snell RS. *Clinical Embryology for Medical Students*. Little, Brown and Company, 1975; 203–48.

Related topic of interest

Bartholin's glands (p. 14)

EPILEPSY AND PREGNANCY

The risk of an epileptic mother having an epileptic baby is about 1:40. Pregnancy itself does not provoke epileptic seizures in pregnancy, but the increased rate of clearance of the anticonvulsants from the circulation. Seizure control in pregnancy is unpredictable, due to the changes in protein binding and metabolism.

It is now generally accepted that most patients with epilepsy can be satisfactorily managed with one drug. The drug of choice is probably carbamazepine. Folic acid is now also widely prescribed because of the associated folate deficiency of patients taking anticonvulsant therapy, thus pre-conceptual counselling is of value.

It is important to monitor the serum anticonvulsant level as the dosage will usually increase during pregnancy although not always. Any change in medication should be made before conception so that seizure control is established with one anticonvulsant drug. Anticonvulsant levels can be monitored in salivary gland secretion.

Associated problems

An increased incidence of vaginal bleeding has been reported which was thought to be due to the effect on uterine contractility and blood coagulation by the commonly used anticonvulsants phenytoin and phenobarbitone.

Seizure frequency will increase in one-third of women during pregnancy, possibly associated with reduced anticonvulsant levels. Fits do not usually affect the fetus.

Placental abruption has a 3-fold increase in epileptic patients, although there is no increase in the rate of placenta praevia.

More serious cases of pre-eclampsia are more common in epileptic patients, although it is often difficult to differentiate between an eclamptic and an epileptic seizure.

Hypoxic signs have been seen in the fetal heart rate following a grand mal seizure, although it is unsure whether this is due to transient hypoxia of the placenta or due to post-ictal apnoea of the mother.

The CTG that is now regularly used both antenatally and during labour can be effected by anticonvulsant therapy, phenobarbitone and valium can cause a non-reactive trace.

It has been shown that there is a 3-fold increase in interventional delivery in the fetus of a patient with epilepsy.

There also appears to be a 3-fold increase in the incidence of term breech presentation in patients who have kept there anticonvulsant levels in the therapeutic levels. The reason is thought to be that the drugs prevent spontaneous version because of its effects on uterine activity. Anticonvulsant therapy is not generally a contraindication to breast feeding.

Congenital anomalies

The incidence of congenital malformations in the offspring of epileptic women receiving anticonvulsants is twice that of the general population. The risks increase with the number of anticonvulsants used.

Various malformations have been reported in infants of epileptic mothers, the most well known being cardiovascular and orofacial. The cardiovascular abnormalities are four times greater than the general population, whereas the orofacial abnormalities are (cleft lip and/or palate) six times more common.

A specific association between neural tube defects and exposure to valproate (1.5%) has been reported. It is thought that the teratogenicity is least with carbamezapine (1% risk of NTD).

Fetal hydantoin syndrome

- Craniofacial anomalies.
- Nail and digital hypoplasia.
- Growth retardation.
- Mental deficiency.
- Genital abnormalities, e.g. hypospadias.

The incidence of this syndrome in infants exposed to the drug *in utero* is 11% with a further 31% showing some features.

Folic acid deficiency is recognized as an unwanted effect of anticonvulsant medication due to hepatic enzyme induction. 5 mg/day of folate is the required suplementation for the epileptic woman.

Epilepsy and contraception

The combined oral contraceptive pill can be safely used, but because of the induction of liver enzymes by certain drugs, 50 µg preparations (Ovran) are sometimes necessary. To ensure efficacy day 21 progesterone can be serially monitored.

The progesterone only pill may have a higher failure rate if the woman is also using liver inducing drugs, so double the dose is advised. Implants and Depo-preparations are unaffected.

Sodium valproate does not affect oral contraceptive efficacy.

Further reading

O'Brien MD, Gilmour-White S. Epilepsy and pregnancy. *British Medical Journal,* 1993; **307:** 492–95.
Robertson IG. Epilepsy in pregnancy. In: Stirrat GM, Beeley L, eds. *Clinics in Obstetrics and Gynaecology,* **13:2,** 365–84.

Related topics of interest

Neonatology (p. 251)
Prenatal diagnosis (p. 281)

EPISIOTOMY

Episiotomy is an obstetric operation in which the perineum is incised during the second stage of labour to increase the area of the pelvic outlet.

Methods

The most commonly performed incision is mediolateral. Alternatives are a midline incision or a 'J'-shaped combination of the two.

Indications

Episiotomy is invariably performed as a prelude to forceps delivery to minimize perineal and vaginal trauma.

1. Maternal. To minimize perineal trauma when the perineum begins to or is about to tear. To minimize the maternal effort at delivery in the presence of maternal disease such as poorly controlled hypertension, cardiac valve anomalies, or where raised intracranial pressure is potentially dangerous such as in the presence of berry aneurysms.

2. Fetal. To facilitate delivery of the fetus in the presence of fetal distress, to minimize trauma to the fetal head and facilitate controlled delivery in premature babies and to minimize trauma to the fetus of the manipulations of assisted breech delivery.

Technique

Adequate analgesia with local or regional anaesthesia is necessary. A scissors cut is made from the posterior fourchette in the midline in the posterolateral direction (mediolateral incision), incising posterior vaginal wall, perineal fibromuscular tissue and skin.

Repair is in layers with an absorbable suture: a continuous suture to the posterior vaginal wall, interrupted sutures to the deep tissues and interrupted or subcuticular sutures to the skin.

Perineal trauma

The perineum is said to tear when the tissues are traumatized at delivery. A first-degree tear involves skin and vaginal epithelium. When the perineal and anal musculature is damaged it is termed a second-degree tear. If the anal or rectal mucosa is torn then a third-degree tear has occurred.

The principles of repair are as for episiotomy, although greater technical difficulties may be encountered with a severe tear. Third-degree tears require careful repair in anatomical layers, from rectal mucosa without and should be undertaken by experienced personnel.

Complications

Haematoma formation, as a result of inadequate haemostasis, predisposes to infection and wound breakdown. This process results in increased pain and delayed healing. Long-term complications arise as a result of increased fibrosis with prolonged pain and dyspareunia.

Poor technique increases the risk of haematoma formation, and may give rise to early wound breakdown in the absence of infection. In addition, long-term complications with fibrosis and skin tag formation, leading to dyspareunia, may also result from poor technique.

Incontinence of flatus and/or faeces may be the result of an inadequately repaired third-degree tear; rarely a permanent colostomy may be required.

Recommended suture material and method. Results from clinical trials indicate that the incidence of short-term pain and analgesic requirements are less when the suture material is polyglycolic acid (Dexon) and the perineal skin is closed using a continuous subcuticular suture. No significant difference in long-term complications has been reported.

Further reading

Grant A. Repair of perineal trauma. In: Chalmers I, Enkin M, Keirse MJNC, eds. *Effective Care in Pregnancy and Childbirth*. Oxford: Oxford University Press, 1989; 1170–81.

Related topics of interest

Analgesia/anaesthesia in labour (p. 163)
Breech (p. 175)
Forceps and ventouse (p. 215)
Perioperative complications in obstetrics and gynaecology (p. 100)
Puerperal sepsis (p. 300)

FETOMATERNAL HAEMORRHAGE AND BLOOD GROUP INCOMPATIBILITY

The human immune system manufactures antibody to neutralize foreign protein (antigen) that it is exposed to. In pregnancy such immunization may occur when fetal red blood cells cross over into the maternal circulation (fetomaternal haemorrhage). Rarely, such an immunization may also occur after an incompatible blood transfusion. The maternally derived antibody will then combine with any further antigenic fetal blood cells that it is exposed to and sequester them in the maternal reticuloendothelial system. In the current and subsequent pregnancies this may result in this maternally derived IgG antibody crossing back over the placenta into the fetal circulation. If the fetus is positive for the antigen in question an antibody-antigen complex is formed on the surface of the fetal red blood cells. This complex results in haemolysis of the fetal red blood cells, leading to erythroblastosis fetalis and haemolytic disease of the newborn. The first pregnancy in which the isoimmunization occurs is generally unaffected, with the severity of effect increasing with increase in the number of pregnancies.

Kleihauer test

The Kleihauer test demonstrates the presence of fetal red blood cells in the maternal circulation. It is the hallmark test of fetomaternal haemorrhage. The adult haemoglobin is acid or alkali eluted from the film, leading to 'ghosting' of the adult haemoglobin cells, whereas fetal haemoglobin, HbF, which is resistant to acid and alkali elution, retains its original colour. It is now recognized that some adults do carry excess amounts of endogenous HbF, and this may lead to confusion as to whether fetomaternal haemorrhage has occurred and to the severity of the haemorrhage. An immunofluorescent technique has been described to distinguish between HbF cells of maternal and fetal origins, and this should be used where there is confusion.

Fetomaternal haemorrhage: causes

(a) 'Silent' or occult haemorrhage, i.e. not clinically detectable abruption – especially second trimester.
- 3–4% risk of isoimmunization.
(b) Antepartum haemorrhage.
(c) Placental abruption.
(d) Transabdominal uterine trauma – iatrogenic and traumatic.
(e) Pre-eclampsia and eclampsia.
(f) Spontaneous vaginal delivery.

(g) Forceps delivery.

(h) Caesarean section.

(i) Manual removal of the placenta.

(j) Multiple birth.

Blood group incompatibility

Maternal and fetal blood group incompatiblity may also result from ABO blood group and non-Rhesus incompatibility. ABO incompatibility results from maternal serum antibody to the fetal red blood cell A or B antigen. This incompatibility is in fact the commonest cause of haemolytic disease of the newborn and erythroblastosis fetalis. More uncommonly other non-ABO and non-Rhesus antigens may lead to haemolytic disease of the newborn, e.g. Kell and Duffy.

Further reading

Whitfield CR. Blood disorders in pregnancy. In: Whitfield CR, ed. *Dewhurst's Textbook of Obstetrics and Gynaecology for Postgraduates*, 4th edn. Oxford: Blackwell Scientific Publications, 1986; 254–76.

Related topics of interest

Immunology of pregnancy (p. 225)
Rhesus disease (p. 311)

FORCEPS AND VENTOUSE

Both instruments are used to expedite vaginal delivery and Wrigley's forceps can be used at LSCS to expedite delivery of the head.

Types of forceps

1. *Outlet forceps.* Wrigley's have a fixed pivot lock and short handles, with a pelvic and a cephalic curve to the blades.

2. *Lift out forceps.* Simpson's are similar to the above but with longer handles so that more traction can be applied.

3. *Rotational forceps.* Kielland's have a sliding lock, a cephalic curve, but only a minimal pelvic curve to enable rotation of the head.

Types of ventouse

1. *Rigid cup.* Including the metal vacuum cups of Malmstrom and Bird.

2. *Soft/flexible cup.* Cone shaped silastic, or disposable plastic.

Indications

- Delay in second stage: commonly 1 hour of active pushing can be associated with malposition, i.e. POP, persistent transverse position.
- Maternal exhaustion with failure of expulsive efforts.
- Maternal compromise: eclampsia/severe pre-eclampsia, intrapartum haemorrhage, cardiac or pulmonary disease.
- Fetal distress: a premature separation of the placenta, cord prolapse at full dilatation.
- The after-coming head of a breech.
- Dural tap after inadvertent placing of the epidural catheter.

Prerequisite requirements for an instrumental delivery

- The cervix must be fully dilated.
- Membranes must be ruptured.
- Position of head and station must be identified – head must be engaged with no more than one-fifth of the head palpable per abdomen.
- No cephalopelvic disproportion.
- Bladder catheterized.

- Adequate analgesia – spinal for rotational forceps delivery.
- Legitimate indication.
- The uterus must be contracting.
- Adequate facilities for neonatal resuscitation.
- Anaesthetist present – all forceps could end with a Caesarean section.

The same conditions apply to the successful use of the ventouse. However the ventouse should not be considered as an easy option when adverse features are present or the position of the fetal head is not known.

Complications

1. Maternal. The perineum and vagina can be damaged, extension of the episiotomy and additional vaginal lacerations can occur during application of the blades and during rotation. The cervix can be damaged during rotational deliveries. Avulsion of the cervix can occur with injudicious placement of the ventouse on a not fully dilated cervix.

Damage to both the bladder and urethra can occur which may result in fistula formation. Urinary complications such as retention and infection can occur. If haematuria is present then continuous bladder drainage should occur for 48 hours after clear urine is present. Pelvic sepsis can also occur. The patient can also be prone to back strain and nerve root or sciatic plexus damage by poor positioning during delivery and also if excessive movement occurs.

2. Fetal. Compression distortion injuries resulting in tears of the tentorium and consequent haemorrhage from the attached veins. Skull fractures can occur and are usually linear and not depressed. Cephalhaematomas are common over the parietal bone and are more common with the use of the ventouse. Jaundice post delivery is also common (more often with the ventouse). Facial nerve palsy can occur by injudicious pressure over it during forceps delivery. Retinal haemorrhages (unknown significance) seem to be more common with the ventouse.

Failed forceps (ventouse) delivery means that the forceps delivery was initiated in the delivery room, but it had to be abandoned in favour of a Caesarean section.

Discusssion

The Royal College of Obstetricians and Gynaecologists advises that the ventouse should be the instrument of first choice for assisted delivery. This is based on evidence from randomized control trials showing reduced maternal trauma without an increase in fetal trauma. It is suggested however, that randomized control trials are not always as objective as they seem.

The vacuum extractor occupies less space and does not have the potential for increasing relative disproportion as forceps do by lying between the fetal skull and side wall.

Traction with a ventouse is linear and allows for rotation of the head to occur on its own, whereas forceps grip the head in four places and control rotation. Forceps approximately double the risk of damaging the anal sphincter and causing bowel symptoms.

The incidence of maternal and fetal trauma are as follows

1. *Instrumental delivery and 3° tear.* 5–40%.

2. *NVD + ventouse.* 35% anal sphincter.
   3% bowel symptoms (flatus, faecal urgency).
   Forceps is double the figures for ventouse.

3. *Pain.* 11% ventouse vs. 17% forceps.

4. *Superficial scalp damage.* 44% ventouse vs. 29–71% forceps.

5. *Cephalohaematoma.* 3.9–13.9% ventouse vs. 2.2–7% forceps.

6. *Retinal haemorrhage.* 34–64% ventouse vs. 16–38% forceps.

Ventouse may require less pain relief, as applying the cap is no more painful than a vaginal examination. The presence of a chinon for 48 hours after delivery can cause maternal concern.

Forceps can be carried out quickly, and in skilled hands there is no difference in morbidity to baby or mother than the ventouse. The big advantage of forceps is its speed, as often an instrumental delivery is required for fetal distress in the second stage. However the rapid application of vacuum significantly reduces the duration of ventouse extraction without compromising safety or efficiency.

Forceps deliveries are associated with a two-fold increase in birth canal trauma.

No discussion of instrumental delivery would be complete without a mention of shoulder dystocia. This occurs when after delivery of the head the shoulders are impacted at the brim. The delay usually occurs because the bi-acromial diameter fails to rotate to enter the transverse diameter of the brim. It can be suspected if there is difficulty in delivering the face and chin and the face is seen to be fat. The incidence is thought to be approximately 1 in 300 deliveries.

This is obviously an obstetric emergency and requires expedient delivery of the fetus. The patient is placed in lithotomy position and the legs flexed further (McRoberts manoeuvre). Anaesthesia may be required. The fetal head is grasped on each side and downward traction is made without rotation. A generous episiotomy is often required. Supra-pubic pressure towards the fetal chest by an assistant to encourage delivery of the anterior shoulder is often necessary, along with fundal pressure and maternal exertion. Once the anterior shoulder is delivered the posterior shoulder follows easily. Rotation of the head may be required to deliver the anterior shoulder. If these actions fail, it may be possible to deliver the posterior shoulder by passing a hand into the sacral hollow and identifying the posterior humerus which is followed to the elbow. This can then be flexed, allowing the wrist to be grasped. Traction sweeps it over the fetal chest to allow delivery of the arm; further traction will convert this shoulder to an anterior position.

If unsuccessful, a symphysiotomy or replacement of the head and subsequent Caesarean section (Zavanelli manoeuvre) can be attempted.

Complications such as brachial plexus injuries, fracture of the clavicle (intentionally or not) and humerus are common; 20% of infants surviving after shoulder dystocia have some form of birth trauma and there is a 30% incidence of long-term neurological complications, including Klumpke's paralysis and Erb's palsy.

Further reading

Drife JO. Choice and instrumental delivery. *British Journal of Obstetrics and Gynaecology,* 1996; **103:** 608–11.

Greis JB, *et al.* Comparison of maternal and fetal effects of vacuum extraction with forceps and caesarean deliveries. *Obstetrics and Gynaecology,* 1981; **57:** 571–7..

Hibbard BM. Forceps delivery. In: Turnbull Sir AC, Chamberlain GC, eds. *Obstetrics,* Edinburgh: Churchill Livingstone, 1991; **56:** 833–48.

Kielland C. The application of forceps to the unrotated head. *Monatsschrift fur Geburtshilffe und Gynakologie,* 1916; **43:** 48–78.

Lim FTH, Holm JP, Schuitemaker NWE, Jansen FH, Hermans J. Stepwise compared with rapid application of vacuum in ventouse extraction procedures. *British Journal of Obstetrics and Gynaecology,* 1997; **104:** 33–6.

O'Grady JP, Gimovsky M. Instrumental delivery: a lost art? In: Studd J, ed. *Progress in Obstetrics and Gynaecology,* 1993; **10:** 183–212.

Roberts L. Shoulder Dystocia.In: Studd J, ed. *Progress in Obstetrics and Gynaecology,* 1994; **11:** 201–16.

Related topics of interest

HOME VERSUS HOSPITAL CONFINEMENT

In the 1920s, 80% of babies were born at home; today the figure is no more than 1%. There is now an increase in the demand for home birth. It is recommended that all Health Authorities have a policy on home confinements. A child, born anywhere, in a situation where his or her life's chances are jeopardized as a result of the birth has recourse to action in law through The Congenital Disabilities (Civil Liability) Act 1976.

Factors causing an increase in home births

(a) Rises in obstetric intervention in labour, especially induction of labour, invasive fetal monitoring, operative vaginal delivery and Caesarean section.

(b) The increasing evidence that such obstetric intervention cannot be justified in the light of maternal and perinatal morbidity and mortality statistics.

(c) The right of women to have a choice in the place of the birth of their baby.

(d) The increasing importance attached to the emotional and psychological well-being of the pregnant woman, her partner, family and baby.

(e) The increase in the number of maternity support groups actively promoting home birth.

Double-figure rates of induction of labour, across the board for all pregnancies, cannot be justified, nor has continuous fetal monitoring been shown to dramatically improve neonatal outcome. Caesarean section rates of greater than 15% are now the norm in many parts of the western world. Factors (c) and (d) above are probably the key to understanding the increased demand for home birth. These factors have been emphasized in the House of Commons Health Committee Report on Maternity Services, and reflected in the responses by the Royal Colleges of Obstetricians and Gynaecologists, Midwives and General Practitioners. There have been a number of recent cases, involving planned domiciliary and hospital confinements, whereby obstetricians have resorted to the Courts to seek judicial consent for emergency Caesarean section, and this is reflected in guidelines published by the RCOG.

Sociology and psychology

The preference for home birth rises with parity, a previous home birth experience and is generally greater than the numbers actually undergoing home confinement. The wish to have a subsequent baby at home after a home birth is of the order of 90%, irrespective of the difficulty of the home confinement, and of those women who have experienced both a hospital and a home birth, 76% prefer the home environment, 15% prefer the hospital, with 9% expressing no particular preference. Most home confinements are associated with the pregnant woman being in control, in her own home, surrounded by a partner, family and attendants (generally a midwife) of her choice, labouring spontaneously, in a non-interventionist atmosphere. Analgesic requirements, episiotomy rates and active management of the third stage rates are lower, breast feeding rates are higher and maternal satisfaction is demonstrably greater. The 1977 Select Committee on Violence in the Family advocated more home deliveries as it facilitates bonding with the newborn and reduces the likelihood of abuse.

Safety

If one excludes obvious high-risk pregnancies that should be delivered in hospital, then home confinement is probably safe. The data are incomplete, but such data as there are would suggest that planned home confinement is no more hazardous than hospital confinement, and may be appreciably safer. A home confinement perinatal mortality rate (PNMR) of 4.1 per 1000 has been quoted, but this does not take into account transfers to hospital of labouring women (about 10% of all planned home births). Calculations, extrapolated from such groups, have shown the PNMR to be of the order of 8 per 1000, which is the same overall range as for many hospital units. It is known that the PNMR of unplanned home births is very high, up to 196.6 per 1000. In the main the women who choose home confinement are a select group, both medically and obstetrically, concentrated in the 25–34 years age range and in the higher social classes, all factors associated with a better maternal and perinatal outcome. In the last triennium there were no maternal mortalities in those women who underwent a home confinement, planned or unplanned. It must be borne in mind that the major unexpected hazards of any birth, fetal distress, cord prolapse, shoulder dystocia, neonatal apnoea, retained placenta and post-partum haemorrhage, are no respecters of geography.

Further reading

Ford PGT. Natural childbirth and home deliveries – medico-legal aspects. In: Chamberlain, G, Orr CJB, Sharp F, eds. *Litigation and Obstetrics and Gynaecology.* Proceedings of the Fourteenth Study Group of the Royal College of Obstetricians and Gynaecologists. London: Royal College of Obstetricians and Gynaecologists, 1985; 301–8.

Milton PJ. Natural childbirth and home deliveries – clinical aspects. In: Chamberlain G, Orr CJB, Sharp F, eds. *Litigation and Obstetrics and Gynaecology.* Proceedings of the Fourteenth Study Group of the Royal College of Obstetricians and Gynaecologists. London, May 1985. London: Royal College of Obstetricians and Gynaecologists, 1985; 279–311.

RCOG Guidelines Ethics. A consideration of the law and ethics in relation to Court-authorised obstetric interventions. RCOG, No 1 April 1994.

Related topics of interest

Post-partum haemorrhage (p. 266)
Report on Confidential Enquiries into Maternal Deaths in the United Kingdom 1991–1993 (p. 309).

HYDROPS FETALIS

Described originally over 100 years ago, its incidence however has remained reasonably stable at 1 in 2–3000 births.

Hydrops fetalis is accumulation of fluid in some or all of the serous cavities in the fetus accompanied by generalized oedema of the skin. The placenta can also be oedematous. It presents usually as polyhydramnios or large for dates uterus. It can present as an intrauterine death associated with oligohydramnios and small for dates. It is associated with anaemia in pregnancy and an increased risk of developing pre-eclampsia. In the presence of a structural abnormality, mortality approaches 100%, in the best scenario rates are about 50%.

In general terms hydrops can occur secondary to anaemia, cardiac failure and a reduction in the osmotic pressure (hypoproteinaemia).

Aetiology

- *Rhesus iso-immunization:* auto-immune hydrops.
- *Cardiac lesions:* Congenital heart block.
- *Chromosomal abnormalities:* Trisomy, Turner's syndrome, triplody.
- *Congenital malformations:* diaphragmatic hernia, post urethral valves.
- *Haematological:* beta-thalassaemia, G-6PD deficiency.
- *Twin-twin transfusion syndrome.*
- *Infections:* TORCH, parvovirus, listeriosis.
- *Placental lesions:* chorioangioma.
- *Umbilical cord lesions:* umbilical vein thrombosis.
- *Maternal conditions:* diabetes mellitus, anaemia.
- *Idiopathic:* accounts for between 15 and 30% of cases.

In the above list, the first cause is the classic auto-immune hydrops, with the remaining causes accounting for the ever increasing number of non-immune hydrops.

Management

1. *Ultrasound.* This should be the first investigation, as it enables the diagnosis to be made. The features seen on a USS are oedema of the scalp, pleural effusions and/or a diaphragmatic hernia, pericardial effusion, ascites associated with increased abdominal circumference, hydrocelles in a male infant, increased liquor pool depth >8 cm, oedema of the placenta.

If the fetus has not had an anomaly scan, it is important to perform this in order to rule out any obvious anomaly that is associated with chromosomal anomalies, e.g. omphalocelle and trisomy 18. Echocardiography and Doppler studies are also useful.

2. *Maternal blood.* Check blood group and antibodies. Take blood cultures if pyrexial, as well as a full blood count. Random blood glucose followed by a GTT may be indicated. Renal and liver function tests should be performed because of the association with PET.

3. *Fetal tests.* Fetal heart rate (CTG) monitoring is indicated, as may be an expert ultrasound of the cardiac anatomy. Fetal blood sampling may be indicated (cordocentesis) to look for an infective cause such as parvovirus, and also to perform chromosomal studies to elucidate the fetal karyotype. Amniocentesis may be performed and is often used in the assessment of rhesus disease.

Treatment This depends on the cause, the severity and the gestation of the fetus and cannot be generalized. In general the prognosis is poor, particularly if fetal movements are reduced.

Further reading

Holzgreve *et al.* Investigation of non-immune hydrops fetalis. *American Journal of Obstetrics and Gynaecology,* 1984; **150:** 805–12.

Related topics of interest

IMMUNOLOGY OF PREGNANCY

The fetus is a foreign tissue graft, or allograft, as it derives half of its genetic material from the father, yet in most pregnancies the maternal immunorejection mechanisms do not cause a failure of the pregnancy.

Systems preventing immunological fetal rejection

(a) Trophoblast lacks detectable expression of class I and II MHC (HLA transplantation) antigens.

(b) Placental 'sink' Fcγ receptors, acting as filters, preferentially bind aggregated or antigen-complexed IgG, formed as a result of the immune reaction between the local fetal antigens and the maternally derived IgG, i.e they sequester them locally in the placental sink.

(c) Unusual class I-like MHC antigen on extravillous cytotrophoblast tissue functions to provide T-cell surveillance of fetal tissue at risk of viral infection and/or for fetal signalling of maternal immunoregulatory responses.

(d) Maternal antibody responses may be altered, the so-called 'blocking antibodies', to influence maternal cell-mediated immunity to the fetus.

(e) Maternal cellular responses may change, e.g. maternal circulating, cytotoxic effector T cells specific for paternally derived lymphocytes, expressed via the fetal intermediary, only occur rarely in a normal pregnancy.

(f) The maternal-fetal interface may act to protect the allograft from infection.

(g) Other factors, e.g progesterone, prostaglandins, interferons and decidual leucocytes (via a suppressor role), may all act in immunoregulatory ways to give a non-specific immunosuppression at maternal-fetal interstices. Transferrin is crucial in the transfer of iron from the mother to the fetus, and it is also essential to the proliferation of any lymphocyte line. The preferential utilization of transferrin by the fetus, for iron uptake, may effectively prevent such proliferation.

Specific conditions

1. Recurrent spontaneous abortion (RSA). An auto-immune explanation for a significant percentage of recurrent miscarriages is held to be explained by the primary antiphospholipid syndrome. It features recurrent miscarriage in association with thrombosis, thrombocytopenia and antiphospholipid antibodies on assay. Antiphospholipid antibodies include lupus anticoagulant and anticardiolipin antibodies. There is a prevalence of antiphospholipid antibodies in 15% of recurrent miscarriage patients compared with 2% in women with no previous history of miscarriage. Current treatment regimes vary, but it is possible that a combination of aspirin and heparin will eventually turn out to be the treatment of choice. In contradistinction immunizing women with paternal or new partner leucocytes, known as immunotherapy, confers no additional benefit on pregnancy outcome, where previously this was thought to be a reasonable treatment.

2. *Systemic lupus erythematosus (SLE)*. This is a multisystem disease relatively common in women of child-bearing age. Its prevalence is 1:700 in white women aged 15–64 years and 1:245 in black women. The diagnosis is based on American Rheumatism Foundation criteria and testing for antinuclear factor and anti-DNA antibodies. SLE pregnancies generally do not affect the long-term SLE prognosis. The pregnancy-related syndrome encompasses thrombotic episodes, thrombocytopenia, IUGR and fetal death. Proteinuria and thrombocytopenia are usually found and can make the differential diagnosis with PET difficult. Most centres report a 5-year survival >95%. Treatment is with aspirin, prednisone and azothiaprine.

3. *Anti-Ro (SS-A) antibody.* This autoantibody is found in 25% of SLE patients and 50% of Sjogren's syndrome patients and may also be found in neonates with the dermatological and heart block manifestations of maternally derived SLE. The congenital heart block is permanent.

4. *Idiopathic thrombocytopenic purpura (ITP).* This is a diagnosis of exclusion, characterized by IgG autoantibodies leading to platelet destruction. They may

cross the placenta and cause transient neonatal thrombocytopenia. Such patients are at risk of haemorrhage at the time of delivery. They may require corticosteroid treatment.

Further reading

De Swiet M. Systemic lupus erythematosus and other connective tissue disorders. In: De Swiet M, ed. *Medical Disorders in Obstetric Practice*, 2nd edn. Oxford: Blackwell Scientific Publications, 1989; 408–25.

Johnson PM. Immunology of pregnancy. In: Turnbull Sir AC, Chamberlain GC, eds. *Obstetrics*. Edinburgh: Churchill Livingstone, 1989; 173–87.

Rai R, Clifford K, Regan L. The modern preventative treatment of recurrent miscarriage. *British Journal of Obstetrics and Gynaecology*, 1996; **103**: 106–110.

Related topics of interest

Fetomaternal haemorrhage and blood group incompatibility (p. 213)
Rhesus disease (p. 311)

INDUCTION OF LABOUR

Induction of labour (IOL) is 'an obstetric procedure designed to pre-empt the natural process of labour by initiating its onset artificially before this occurs spontaneously', and in pragmatic terms it also implies a successful completion of labour. Labour itself may be defined as the onset of increasingly more frequent, sustained and painful uterine contractions, accompanied by descent of the presenting part and dilatation of the uterine cervix. Two hundred years ago Denman induced labour, preterm, by amniotomy, to avoid cephalopelvic disproportion, and in 1909 William Blair Bell introduced oxytocin into clinical practice.

Physiology

The main anatomical constituents in labour are the pituitary, uterus, decidua, placenta, amniotic membranes, amniotic fluid, fetus and cervix. It is postulated that it is an increase in the concentration of free calcium ions within the intracellular sarcoplasmic reticulum of the uterine smooth muscle that promotes actin and myosin filament activity, thereby leading to uterine contractility. Prostaglandins (PGs), especially $PGF_2\alpha$, stimulate the release of calcium ions from the sarcoplasmic reticulum. They probably act via a second messenger at the amniotic membrane level (which are a rich source of arachidonic acid, the main PG precursor), and also to sensitize the myometrium to oxytocin. Unlike PGs, oxytocin is not involved in the primary initiation of labour, and the pregnant uterus is only fully sensitive to oxytocin in late pregnancy and secondary to the PG rise in late pregnancy. There is also a PG surge in the third stage of labour, which is highly likely to contribute to the expulsion of the placenta and membranes, a factor made use of in the face of a severe PPH, when intramyometrial PGs are given. Other important contributory hormones include oestrogen, progesterone (which is generally held to be tocolytic via two mechanisms: inactivation by progesterone dehydrogenase of fetal kidney-derived PGs and stimulation by progesterone or myometrial sarcoplasmic reticulum uptake of calcium ions), fetal cortisol (which has been shown to be crucial to the initiation of labour in the pregnant sheep), arginine vasopressin, adenyl cyclase, catecholamines, corticosteroids, corticotrophin, relaxin, inhibin, cAMP and phospholipase C.

The cervix

The uterine cervix is very important in labour, going from a closed sphincter, via 'ripening' and effacement, to an open conduit for labour and delivery. This is achieved by a decrease in the amount of, and modification of, the cervical connective tissue, leading to a massive increase in compliance, which in turn allows dilatation to occur. PGs are vital to this process. Vaginal assessment of the cervix, using a quantitative method such as the Bishop score, is currently the best available way of assessing the ease of induction of labour. Bishop found a clear inverse relationship between the cervical score and the time until onset of spontaneous labour, i.e. the lower the score the greater the interval to onset of labour. It must be appreciated that labour is not a sudden event, rather it is the culmination of a gradual process, 'prelabour', evolving over a period of weeks. The critical events of 'prelabour' are a gradual increase in myometrial contractility (generally >35/40), and a change in the shape and compliance of the cervix known as 'ripening'. Natural labour in a primapara proceeds at a rate of 1.3 cm/h cervical dilatation, with a mean first stage of 5.6 hours and with 99% being delivered within 10 hours from time of admission.

Prostaglandins

Currently, the most successful regimen is vaginal PGE_2 2 mg followed by amniotomy 4–6 hours later followed by IV oxytocin (15 IU in 500 ml of dextrose saline, commenced at 2 d.p.m., increasing by increments to a maximum of 96 d.p.m. = 48 mU/min) 1–4 hours later. This results in >95% of women being brought into labour and a 12% Caesarean section rate, with only 2–5% of sections being the result of a failure to establish labour. Vaginal PGs, followed by repeat vaginal PGs to avoid IV oxytocin, are less successful than the above regimen. Tumultuous rapid labour is uncommon. Analgesic requirements and the rate of PPH are diminished compared with other forms of induction. Meta-analysis has shown PGs to be safe when administered to those women with ruptured membranes who require augmentation of labour, and those undergoing a 'trial of scar' or induction with a twin pregnancy are also safe. In the author's experience intrauterine fetal death induction of labour and delivery are now probably best initiated using mifepristone 600 mgm at time zero, and misoprostol, 400–800 mgm PV at 48 hours and thereafter misoprostol 600 mgm orally at 51, 54 and 57 hours. The role of induction of labour in the singleton breech pregnancy is untested by scientific trial at the time of writing.

Problems

There are no significant differences between the umbilical cord gases of babies whose mothers have been induced with PGs and those whose mothers are labouring spontaneously. Continuous fetal monitoring is not indicated with routine induction of labour cases, although it is wise to perform a 20 minute cardiotocograph after administration of PGs. There are a few reports of intrauterine fetal death after PGs and one of abruption. There is a 1% risk of uterine overstimulation and a 0.2% risk of uterine hypertonus leading to a sustained tetanic contraction necessitating immediate delivery by section or urgent tocolysis. These figures equal the rate of such events in spontaneous-onset labours, i.e. there is no significant difference.

The fetus and neonate

Prostaglandins cross into the fetal circulation, but there is no evidence that this has any adverse physiological outcome, including *in utero* closure of the ductus arteriosus. Babies delivered after induction show no adverse outcome when followed up for 12 or 36 months. Prostaglandins, because of their steroid effects, reduce neonatal hyperbilirubinaemia, and their use has reduced the incidence of neonatal (and maternal) hyponatraemia, a side-effect of sustained, high-dose oxytocic infusions.

Further reading

Calder A. Induction and augmentation of labour. In: Turnbull Sir AC, Chamberlain GC, eds. *Obstetrics*. Edinburgh: Churchill Livingstone, 1989; 823–32.

Turnbull AC, Lopez Bernal A. Physiology and biochemistry of labour. In: Turnbull Sir AC, Chamberlain GC, eds. *Obstetrics*. Edinburgh: Churchill Livingstone, 1989; 701–12.

Related topics of interest

INFECTION IN PREGNANCY

Infection has been a major cause of maternal and fetal mortality and, although the outcome has dramatically improved with the advent of antibiotic therapy, infection remains a major health hazard for mother and baby.

Infections can be broadly divided into those which have a predilection for the pregnant woman and those which affect the fetus, either by transplacental transmission *in utero* or by direct infection via the lower genital tract during parturition.

Fever in early pregnancy can cause abortion, and in later pregnancy may lead to premature labour. Therefore any infection associated with a significant pyrexia may carry a risk to the fetus.

Maternal infection

Pregnancy predisposes to certain infections, notably of the urinary system and lower genital tract.

Untreated UTI predisposes to premature labour, and repeated infection may cause renal impairment.

The normal vaginal flora is affected by the hormonal changes in pregnancy, resulting in an increase in candidiasis, particularly in women with gestational diabetes and after treatment with antibiotics. Overall the frequency in pregnancy is of the order of 16%.

Potential pathogens may colonize the vagina and are related to the development of chorioamnionitis and puerperal sepsis. The beta-haemolytic streptococcus is a common pathogen in this situation, and is present in about 15% of pregnant women.

Fetal infection

Certain infective agents cross the placenta and lead to fetal death, abortion or to the development of congenital anomalies.

Maternal symptoms may be minor, leading to a delay in diagnosis.

Direct transmission to the fetus of pathogens colonizing the lower genital tract of the mother may occur at delivery. The resulting illness is more severe because of the immaturity of the fetal immune system.

1. Transplacental infection. Rubella causes few or no symptoms in the pregnant woman, who may only have a mild rash. Fetal effects may cause abortion or result in congenital cardiac anomalies, deafness, cataract or less commonly mental retardation and hepatic impairment.

The more severe consequences result from infection in early pregnancy, with deafness the common result of later infection.

Diagnosis is on serological grounds and termination is offered for proven infection before 17 weeks' gestation. The incidence is greatly reduced by prophylactic immunization; currently all babies are offered inoculation. Conversely, the success of the immunization programme has reduced the level of immunity which arises after natural infection which has resulted in infection of immune patients.

All pregnant women should have rubella serology at booking.

Cytomegalovirus is the commonest congenital infection in the UK (200–300 cases per annum). It is characterized by mental retardation, microcephaly, hydrocephalus, hepatosplenomegaly and petechiae. The mortality is 20% in clinically apparent congenital disease. Less than 5% of infected babies develop manifestations of the disease.

Immune mothers may suffer reinfection, causing difficulty in diagnosis and formulating a policy for screening and giving advice regarding termination.

Toxoplasmosis, which results from the ingestion of a protozoon found in inadequately cooked meat and cat faeces, causes a non-specific infection characterized by lymphadenopathy and lethargy.

Fetal infection results in abortion or congenital cerebral, ocular and aural (deafness) anomalies.

More severe effects are associated with infection earlier in pregnancy. In the UK about 2 in 1000 babies is infected, but only 6 babies per year on average show signs of congenital infection at birth.

Currently screening is not recommended. (RCOG working party, 1992).

Listeria monocytogenes, a Gram-positive rod, is widely prevalent in inadequately stored food such as soft cheese, cook-chill meals and pre-prepared salad. Typically causing a mild biphasic and non-specific maternal illness, it is associated with premature delivery of an infant with respiratory distress, liver impairment and neurological problems. Antibiotic therapy is indicated if maternal blood cultures are positive.

Meconium staining of the liquor in premature labour is suggestive of listeriosis.

Varicella zoster virus crosses the placenta, but significant neonatal effects are uncommon. The most dangerous period to contract the infection is in the few days before delivery, before maternal effects are apparent and before maternal transmission of antibody can occur. In this situation infection may cause neonatal pneumonia, which carries a high (30%) mortality. Affected neonates are given zoster immunoglobulin as soon as possible.

Parvovirus is a common infection occurring in epidemics, 50% of all adults are susceptible. Fetal transmission occurs in 30%. Manifestations are anaemia and hydrops, of which 50% reduce spontaneously.

2. Direct transmission. Chlamydia trachomatis and *Neisseria gonorrhea* are both associated with ocular infection which may lead to blindness if appropriate treatment is delayed.

Herpes simplex virus causes generalized neonatal infection, involving CNS, liver, lungs and eyes. Mortality is high and the risk of infection during delivery if the mother has a primary infection is 50%.

The risk is significantly lower in secondary attacks. Caesarean section is recommended if there is clinical evidence of genital herpes unless the membranes have been ruptured for 4 hours or more.

Evidence suggests that antenatal screening of at-risk groups by repeated vaginal swabs is unhelpful and should be abandoned.

3. Other infections. The neonate is at particular risk in certain situations because of the immaturity of its immune system.

Mothers who have a chronic infection may transmit this to the neonate. The most important examples of this type of infection are hepatitis B and AIDS.

Hepatitis B virus can induce a carrier state, which accounts for a prevalence of about 200 million worldwide. The presence of the hepatitis e antigen carries a greater risk of transmission from mother to fetus; antenatal serology is appropriate in high-risk women such as intravenous drug abusers.

Spread is via infected blood and the perinatal period is one of particularly high risk. Maternal antibody may also be transmitted to the fetus but should disappear by 9 months of age. Persistent antibody suggests an infected baby.

At-risk babies are given both active and passive immunization at birth. This should result in a decrease in the incidence of the disease worldwide.

HIV infection may be transplacental, the risk being estimated at 25%. This is reduced to 8% by active treatment of HIV positive women and their neonates with zidovudine. The neonate is also at risk from infected maternal blood.

Antibody testing of neonates is of limited value as antibody is acquired from the mother but persistently elevated antibody levels suggest infection. The virus is also present in breast milk and HIV-positive mothers should be advised against breast feeding.

HIV-positive mothers may be offered termination of pregnancy, although pregnancy does not appear to accelerate the course of the disease. The risks to the fetus are those of growth retardation and premature delivery.

Further reading

Hurley Dame R. Fever and infectious diseases. In: De Swiet M, ed. *Medical Disorders in Obstetric Practice*, 2nd edn. Oxford: Blackwell Scientific Publications, 1989: 775–96.

MacLean AB, ed. *Clinical Infection in Obstetrics and Gynaecology*. Oxford: Blackwell Scientific Publications, 1990.

Thornton J, Onwude J. Screening for congenital infection in pregnancy. In: Studd J, ed. *Progress in Obstetrics and Gynaecology,* Vol. 11. Edinburgh: Churchill Livingstone, 1994; 23–37.

Wang E, Small F. Infection in pregnancy. In: Chalmers I, Enkin M, Keirse MJNC, eds. *Effective Care in Pregnancy and Childbirth*, Vol. 1. Oxford: Oxford University Press, 1989: 534–64.

Related topics of interest

INTRAUTERINE DEATH

Almost 1% of women entering the second half of their pregnancy will suffer the loss of their baby.

Diagnosis

The absence of fetal heart sounds, lack of fetal movements and regression of uterine size. Doppler apparatus is useful in picking up the fetal heart, but care should be taken to avoid mistaking transmitted maternal pulsation for a slow fetal heart.

Ultrasound will show an absent fetal heart echo, skull collapse, poorly visualized midline falx, retraction of brain tissue, empty fetal bladder and a non-filled aorta. It may be helpful to show the women the findings as some women may report movements hours after the diagnosis is made.

Plain radiological signs are overlapping of the fetal skull bones (Spalding's sign) or gas in the fetal circulation (Robert's sign) were pathognamonic.

An attempt should always be made to elucidate the cause.

Associated problems

1. *Infection.* While membranes remain intact the chances of infection are negligible.

2. *Maternal distress.* No evidence that hasty induction and delivery lessens parental anguish.

3. *Coagulopathy* can occur after 16 weeks' gestation, but only when the dead fetus has been retained *in utero* for more than 4 weeks. Fibrinogen falls at a rate of 50 mg/dl per week, but is unlikely to cause a bleeding tendency until its level has fallen below 100 mg/dl. It is also associated with a rise in FDP and a fall in platelets. The coagulopathy is thought to be a result of fibrinogen consumption following the release of thromboplastin from the retained products. It is interesting however that only 10% of patients will remain undelivered after 3 weeks if left entirely alone. However if a conservative approach is taken fibrinogen levels, FDP and platelets should be measured weekly.

Investigations

These should be laid down as a protocol and followed for all cases of intrauterine death:

1. Maternal

- FBC.
- Group and antibodies, Kleihauer.
- TORCH, listeria and parvovirus antibodies, Wasserman reaction (WR).
- Glycosylated Hb and random blood glucose.
- U&Es, LFTs, TFTs.
- Maternal and paternal karyotype if fetus abnormal.
- Clotting studies if fetal death >3 weeks.
- Anticardiolipin antibodies and lupus anticoagulant.

2. Fetal

- Post mortem examination.
- X-ray if no consent obtained, with weighing, measuring and an external photo.
- Histology, bacteriology and virology of placenta.
- Genetic examination of placental tissue and fetal skin/blood.
- Cord blood/cardiac blood, e.g. TORCH, cultures, IgM, ABO + rhesus.

Management

Vaginal delivery should be the aim unless specific indications for abdominal delivery are present. Induction of labour with prostaglandins is performed. Two commonly used preparations are:

- *Misoprostol* (PGE_1 analogue) which can be given orally.
- *Gemeprost* (PGE_1 analogue) which can be given vaginally.

Currently advised regimes

- Mifepristone 600 mg orally, followed 36–48 hours later with 1mg gemeprost every 3 hours (max 5 pessaries).
- Mifepristone 200 mg orally, followed 36–48 hours later by 800 µg misoprostol vaginally then 400 µg misoprostol orally, 3 hourly (max 4 oral doses).
- Mifepristone 200 mg orally, followed 36 hours later by 1mg gemeprost vaginally every 6 hours.

Side effects of prostaglandins are a rise in temperature, tachycardia, GIT symptoms, vomiting and diarrhoea. Mifepristone (RU486) in doses 200–600 mg,

24–48 hours prior to prostaglandins, reduces the induction to abortion time by 50%.

In the past intra-amniotic solutions of hypertonic saline (associated with abruption), hypertonic glucose (associated with infectious morbidity) and hypertonic urea have been used. Intra- and extra-amniotic prostaglandin have been used, and also oxytocin.

Twin pregnancy with single fetal death is a difficult problem to manage. Expectant management is advised for the demise of one fetus after 20 weeks gestation. Incidence 0.5–7% has been reported. There needs to be close maternal and fetal monitoring.

There are very few reasons for abdominal delivery in the presence of fetal death:

- Known major degree of placenta praevia.
- Severe CPD where crushing base fetal skull necessary for delivery.
- Previous classical Caesarean section.
- >2 LSCS.
- Incipient uterine rupture or if rupture suspected.

There are a number of relative indications such as a transverse lie or shoulder presentation in advanced labour with ruptured membranes where the alternative is a destructive operation rarely used in modern obstetric practice.

It is very important that documentation of events surrounding an IUD and co-ordination of the investigations which follow should rest with the obstetrician who has admitted the patient; with this in mind most units will have a protocol to follow. It is important that proper puerperal care such as suppression of lactation with bromocriptine or carbergoline (long acting dopamine agonist) and careful bereavement support is offered to the mother after delivery. A follow-up appointment should be made – possibly a domiciliary visit within 6 weeks.

Further reading

Fox R, Pillai M, Porter H, Gill G. Management of late fetal death; a guide to comprehensive care. *British Journal of Obstetrics and Gynaecology,* 1997; **104:** 4–10.

Tindall VR, Reid GD. The management of intrauterine death. In: *Progress in Obstetics and Gynaecology,* Vol 7. Edinburgh: Churchill Livingstone, 1989; **13:** 199–216.

Related topics of interest

Biophysical profile – assessing the at risk fetus (p. 172)
Monitoring in labour (p. 245)
Rhesus disease (p. 311)

INTRAUTERINE GROWTH RETARDATION

Perinatal mortality correlates closely with birthweight and is higher in the small-for-dates or growth retarded fetus. The growth retarded fetus is also likely to be delivered prematurely, suffer from fetal distress or perinatal asphyxia and can result in a stillbirth. The neonate who is growth retarded has significant morbidity due to hypoglycaemia, polycythaemia, hyperbilirubinaemia or to the asphyxia before and during birth.

Intrauterine growth retardation (IUGR) is a general term describing infants whose birthweight is likely to fall below the 10th percentile for gestational age and sex.

Causes

1. *Medical complications*, e.g. pre-eclampsia.

2. *Socio-economic factors*, e.g. malnutrition.

3. *Fetal problems*, e.g. multiple births.

4. *Abnormalities of placenta*, e.g. placenta praevia.

Diagnosis

Diagnosis is made clinically and by the aid of ultrasound. Formerly, abdominal palpation was used; however, this is a less than effective method of determining IUGR. The use of symphysial-fundal height in centimetres (± 3 cm) improves the detection rate for IUGR fetuses but the sensitivity (between 70–88%) and specificity are still poor although better than palpation alone.

Ultrasound scanning is the method of choice. An anomaly scan at 18 weeks to check dates and fetal morphology followed by a second scan in the third trimester for growth offers the highest detection rates for IUGR.

The importance of ultrasound is firstly in the accurate assessment of fetal gestation. It is possible to diagnose an intrauterine gestation sac as early as 5 weeks using a vaginal probe and a fetal heart at 6 weeks. A crown rump length is very accurate from 6 to 12 weeks (estimate error of ± 3.5 days) following which it is possible to determine a bi-parietal diameter, although reliably from 14 weeks (the error before 20 weeks being about 1 week ranging to 3 weeks when performed after 34 weeks). Fetal abdominal circumference is used to estimate fetal weight and weight gain. The measurement is taken by measuring the skin circumference at a plane passing perpendicular to the long axis of the fetus at the level of the intrahepatic portion of the umbilical vein.

The majority of IUGR fetuses (70%) are, in fact normal small fetuses. When the fetal abdomen is small but the BPD is appropriate then the fetus has 'asymmetrical' growth retardation due to an extrinsic cause, e.g. pre-eclampsia. However when both measurements are small and 'symmetrical', IUGR has occurred and can be associated with an intrinsic cause, e.g. Trisomy 21.

Ultrasound must be used for assessing fetal size, as fewer than 40% of growth retarded fetuses are detected by clinical examination alone.

Management

Once a diagnosis has been made, it is important to rule out any intrinsic fetal problem such as renal agenesis or a chromosomal abnormality (more common in symmetrical growth retardation); therefore cordocentesis may be indicated to obtain a karyotype. Extrinsic factors should be minimized, for example the mother should stop smoking and pre-eclampsia or other medical problems, should be treated. If placenta praevia is found, then rest is important.

Fetal growth should be monitored by fortnightly ultrasound scans purely for growth, although it may be necessary to perform regular biophysical profiles in the severely compromized infant, as well as Doppler studies of the utero-placental blood flow and cord resistance index. The aim is to reach 37 weeks gestation if possible and then to expedite delivery. In the severely growth-retarded fetus, many clinicians will opt for delivery by LSCS, because of the lack of fetal reserve for a labour.

Further reading

Campbell S, Wilkin D. Ultrasonic measurement of the fetal abdominal circumference in the estimation of fetal weight. *British Journal of Obstetrics and Gynaecology*, 1975; **83:** 689.

Manning FA, Menticoglou S, Harman S. Fetal assessment by biophysical methods: Ultrasound. In: Turnbull Sir AC, Chamberlain GC, eds. *Obstetrics,* Edinburgh: Churchill Livingstone, 1989; **27:** 383–98.

Related topics of interest

MIDWIFERY

A midwife is defined by the International Confederation of Midwives and the International Federation of Gynaecologists and Obstetricians, following amendment of the World Health Organization (WHO) criteria, as a person who, having been regularly admitted to a midwifery education programme, duly recognized in the country in which it is located, has successfully completed the prescribed course of studies in midwifery and has acquired the requisite qualifications to be registered and/or legally licensed to practice midwifery.

Attributes of a midwife

Midwives must be able to give the necessary supervision, care and advice to women during pregnancy, labour and the puerperium, to conduct deliveries on their own and to care for the newborn and the infant. This care includes preventive measures, the detection of abnormal conditions in mother and child, the procurement of medical assistance and the execution of emergency measures in the absence of medical help. Midwives have an important task in health counselling and education, not only of patients, but also of family and community. The work should involve antenatal education and preparation for parenthood and extends to certain areas of gynaecology, family planning and child care. Midwives may practice in hospitals, clinics, health units, domiciliary conditions or in any other service.

Today there are more than 35 000 registered midwives in the United Kingdom. They act within a set of Midwives Rules, Code of Practice and a Code of Professional Conduct as defined by the United Kingdom Central Council for Nursing, Midwifery and Health Visiting. These are legally expressed in documents known as Statutory Instruments and cover many topics, including age and educational requirements for entry to midwifery courses, programmes of education, examinations, notification of intention to practice, responsibility and sphere of practice, administration of medicines and analgesics, record-keeping, liaison with other medical personnel, definition of an emergency, activities of a midwife, hospital practice, home confinements and notification of a maternal death, stillbirth or neonatal death.

Further reading

Cowell B, Wainwright D. *Behind The Blue Door. The History of the Royal College of Midwives*, 1881–1981. London: Bailliere Tindall, 1981.

A Midwife's Code of Practice, Midwives Rules, Code of Professional Conduct. UKCC, March 1991, and June 1992.

Related topic of interest

Home versus hospital confinement (p. 220)

MONITORING IN LABOUR

Fetal monitoring

The aim of fetal monitoring in labour is to detect signs of hypoxia in the fetus such that, where applicable, delivery may be expedited before a state of serious compromise is reached.

The ideal method should be accurate, non-invasive and unintrusive to the labouring woman. In the absence of such a method, the available monitoring techniques are applied in relation to the degree of risk in each individual labour.

The hypoxic fetus may exhibit signs of distress; the heart rate may be abnormally high or low, there may be a lack of baseline variability of the heart rate and there may be decelerations in the heart rate which are not synchronous with a uterine contraction. These signs may be accompanied by the passage of meconium.

Low-risk labour

When labour involves little risk to the fetus and a multiparous woman with no relevant medical or obstetric history and no antenatal problems, labouring spontaneously at term with a singleton fetus and progressing normally without epidural analgesia, then minimal intervention in terms of monitoring is required.

It has been shown in a large study from Dublin that intermittent auscultation of the fetal heart rate with a Pinard fetal stethoscope by an experienced midwife is as safe in terms of the degree of fetal hypoxia and subsequent morbidity as is continuous external cardiotocography.

In general, it is recommended that a CTG is taken on admission to the labour ward for a duration of 30 minutes and repeated at 4-hourly intervals, with intermittent auscultation in the interim.

Evidence of hypoxia obtained by the above methods, the passage of meconium, vaginal bleeding or the need for obstetric intervention (such as augmentation of slow labour with intravenous syntocinon) will convert the labour into a high-risk one.

High-risk labour

Classification of labour as high risk depends on factors such as age and parity, medical and obstetric history, antenatal complications such as multiple pregnancy, vaginal bleeding, hypertension, proteinuria, IUGR, and intrapartum problems such as premature labour, induced labour, slow progress or fetal distress. There may be passage of meconium or blood without obvious fetal distress.

In high-risk labour continuous CTG recording is employed, with internal tocography using a fetal scalp electrode as the more accurate method.

In its prediction of fetal hypoxia the CTG has a low false-positive rate but a high false-negative rate. In order to minimize unnecessary intervention a more accurate estimation of hypoxia is required. In this situation a fetal scalp capillary blood sample is taken and the pH and blood gases analysed.

A pH value below 7.30 is suggestive of hypoxia, but interpretation of pH values must take account of the stage of labour: pH falls by 0.016 U/h in the first stage and by 0.12 U/h in the second stage.

The correlation between CTG and fetal blood sampling is only 53% between the most ominous CTG pattern, that of a complicated baseline tachycardia, and a hypoxic pH reading.

Results of fetal pulse oximetry have proved difficult to interpret with significant reductions in oxygen saturation having little effect on the fetus. Analysis of the fetal ECG has not been shown to be useful in the clinical setting.

Maternal monitoring

The mother's progress in labour is monitored with a partogram. High-risk situations include pre-eclampsia and epidural analgesia, when frequent estimations of blood pressure are necessary, and the administration of intravenous syntocinon to induce or augment labour.

Uterine activity

A measured dose of intravenous syntocinon, with incremental increases at 15 minute intervals, is delivered via a Cardiff pump. In situations where it is desirable to monitor the pressure of uterine contractions, such as in augmented labour in a woman with a lower segment Caesarean section scar or when the recommended maximum dose of syntocinon is to be increased, then an intrauterine pressure catheter may be required.

The catheter, with a pressure transducer at its tip, is inserted into the uterine cavity beside the fetus. The maximum pressures to be generated are decided upon (e.g. up to 1200 kPa/15 min in the presence of a scar on the uterus and 1800 kPa/15 min with no scar) and syntocinon is administered accordingly.

The rate of dilatation of the cervix does not always correlate with intrauterine pressure and measurement of head-cervix force may be of greater clinical relevance.

Further reading

Beard RW, Filshie GM, Knight CA, Roberts GM. The significance of the changes in the continuous fetal heart rate in the first stage of labour. *Journal of Obstetrics and Gynaecology of the British Commonwealth,* 1971; **78:** 865–81.

Francis JG, Turnbull AC, Thomas FF. Automatic oxytocin infusion equipment for induction of labour. *Journal of Obstetrics and Gynaecology of the British Commonwealth,* 1970; **77:** 594–602.

Macdonald D, Grant A, Sheridan-Pereira M, Boylan P, Chalmers I. The Dublin randomised controlled trial of intrapartum fetal heart rate monitoring. *American Journal of Obstetrics and Gynecology,* 1985; **152:** 524–39.

Steer PJ. Intrapartum Monitoring. In: Studd J, ed. *Progress in Obstetrics and Gynaecology,* Vol. 11. Edinburgh: Churchill Livingstone, 1994; 183–200.

Related topics of interest

MULTIPLE PREGNANCY

Twin pregnancy occurs in about 1 in 80 spontaneous conceptions in the UK. Higher multiples follow Hellin's law. The incidence of higher multiples is reduced by a higher spontaneous abortion rate but is increased as a result of assisted conception techniques.

The incidence of multiple pregnancy is increased with increasing maternal age and a family history of multiple pregnancy.

Physiology

The physiological changes of pregnancy are exaggerated in multiple pregnancy, notably an increase in plasma volume, a lesser increase in red cell mass, with a consequent tendency to anaemia, increased glomerular filtration rate and an increase in pregnancy-related hormones and placental proteins. There is a decreased tolerance to a blood glucose load, tending to the development of gestational diabetes.

Complications

Most pregnancy-related problems are commoner and more severe in multiple pregnancy. The diagnosis may be suspected by exaggerated symptoms of early pregnancy, particularly nausea and vomiting.

Anaemia is commoner, as is gestational diabetes, pre-eclampsia, preterm labour, intrauterine growth retardation and polyhydramnios. Recent studies suggest no great increase in the incidence of antepartum haemorrhage. Twin-twin transfusion syndrome occurs in 5–15% of twin pregnancies and is commoner in monozygotic, monochorionic twins. If acute, the syndrome has a high mortality of 79–100% at 18–26 weeks.

Other pregnancy-related symptoms may cause significant distress, e.g. heartburn, constipation, backache, tiredness and discomfort from haemorrhoids.

Antenatal care

Patients are seen frequently in the antenatal clinic; iron and folate supplements are routinely prescribed. Blood pressure and fetal growth are regularly monitored, with frequent ultrasound scans in later pregnancy.

Amnionicity and chorionicity may be determined by ultrasound in skilled hands and amniocentesis of separate sacs may be performed after appropriate counselling.

For triplet and quad pregnancies consideration is given to cervical cerclage and prophylactic beta-adrenergic agents such as salbutamol to reduce the incidence of prematurity. These patients are usually admitted in the third trimester for bed rest.

Management of labour

Twins may deliver vaginally. The labour should be supervised by an experienced obstetrician with an anaesthetist present and facilities for emergency Caesarean section and expert neonatal care readily available.

Elective Caesarean section may be considered if there is a malpresentation of the first twin, or if maternal or fetal circumstances warrant.

Elective Caesarean section is the preferred mode of delivery for triplets and higher multiples.

Perinatal mortality

For twins and triplets the perinatal mortality rate is about five times that of singleton births. The main aetiological factor is prematurity.

Rare causes of twin mortality include locked and conjoined twins.

The second and third triplets are at greater risk, with a delay in delivery of 5 minutes after the birth of the first triplet being significant. The maturity of the triplets is of greater prognostic significance than their size.

Further reading

Crowther CA, Multiple pregnancy including delivery. In: James DK, Steer PJ, Weiner CP, Gonik B, eds. *High Risk Pregnancy Management Options*. London: WB Saunders, 1994; 137–49.

Daw E. Triplet pregnancy. In: Studd J, ed. *Progress in Obstetrics and Gynaecology*, Vol. 6. Edinburgh: Churchill Livingstone, 1987: 119–31.

MacGillivray I. Multiple pregnancy. In: Turnbull Sir AC, Chamberlain GC, eds. *Obstetrics*. Edinburgh: Churchill Livingstone, 1989: 493–502.

Related topics of interest

NEONATOLOGY

The neonate at delivery is physiologically forced, owing to the removal of the placental system, to adopt an adult circulation and respiratory pattern. Birth is a stressful process, even for the well grown and morphologically normal term fetus. Resuscitation may be necessary if the neonate fails to gasp, expand the lungs or initiate a continuing respiratory pattern, or is cyanotic, bradycardic or apparently stillborn. Assessment of such problems is immediately available in the form of umbilical cord gases and the Apgar score, named after an American paediatrician, Virginia Apgar; the higher the score, the 'better' the state of the neonate. The Apgar score considers five parameters – respiratory effort, reflex irritability, muscle tone, heart rate and colour – scoring each out of 0, 1 or 2 at 1 minute and 5 minutes of age.

Causes of low Apgar scores   Causes include maternal sedation, drugs and anaesthesia, maternal disease such as diabetes, prolonged labour, intrauterine asphyxia (from whatever cause), prematurity, traumatic operative delivery (including intracerebral haemorrhage), congenital anomaly (especially cardiac, pulmonary, neurological and gastrointestinal), chromosomal abnormality, meconium aspiration, infection, growth retardation and respiratory distress syndrome (RDS; also known as hyaline membrane disease).

Resuscitation   (a) All babies at birth should be handled gently, wrapped and kept warm after the cord is clamped, and if 'flat' placed on a resuscitation trolley with a good light and a source of radiant heat.

(b) A pale or blue floppy infant at birth is in need of immediate, active resuscitation.

(c) The neonatal heart rate and respiratory pattern are the key features. Initial manoeuvres should include chest and cardiac auscultation, in conjunction with careful and gentle low-pressure suction of the mouth and oropharynx and trachea, ideally using a laryngoscope to obtain direct vision.

(d) Meconium-stained liquor must be taken seriously, and meconium aspiration considered in any labour complicated by meconium and a neonate with respiratory problems.

(e) Facial oxygen delivered through a face mask and bag may be all that is required to establish normal respiration and circulation, but endotracheal intubation may be required – at a rate of 30–40/min, for 1 second, at a pressure of <30 cm H_2O, avoiding overinflation.

(f) If the neonate remains 'flat' after this, consider why, but institute cardiac massage, adrenaline, and correction of the acidosis that will by now have occurred. Think of pleural effusion or pneumothoraces that may need tapping, or shock, sepsis and bleeding, and commence plasma infusion.

(g) The decision to stop resuscitation must be taken by the most senior member of the paediatric team present.

Common problems

Jaundice (bilirubin >85 µmol/l) is relatively common in the newborn. It may be physiological owing to a delay in hepatocyte function in a normal infant, secondary to an increased red cell mass breakdown as in the Rhesus isoimmunized infant, the infant receiving drugs that impair induction of glucuronyl transferase activity or in the preterm infant. The bilirubin requires serial assay in the jaundiced infant, and if it is present in the first 24 hours of life, persists for more than a week or rises above 200 µmol/l then action in the form of phototherapy (conversion of bilirubin into harmless pigments by UV light) and rarely exchange transfusion should remedy it. Kernicterus is a serious form of brain damage (yellow staining of the basal ganglia with histological evidence of neuronal damage) seen in the severely jaundiced baby when the bilirubin is >340 µmol/l.

RDS maybe diagnosed by clinical examination or radiology. The essential features necessary for the diagnosis include tachypnoea, grunting, intercostal recession (all within 4 hours of birth), and the need for additional oxygen to be delivered to the infant within 24 hours of birth. Radiology may show patchy atelectasis, with small volume, hyperaemic lung fields, lymphatic dilatation and hyaline membranes. The generalized reticulogranular opacity of the lungs is often described as being of a 'ground glass' appearance. The disease is primarily seen in the preterm infant (the prevalence is more than 30% at 28 weeks' gestation), but may occur in the diabetic and the term infant. The frequency in term infants is 0.01%. Treatment in moderate and severe cases is with endotracheal intubation and ventilation, and recently artificial surfactant has shown to be of real benefit in a number of international, multicentre trials. Complications of the disease include pulmonary interstitial emphysema, pneumothorax, persistent fetal circulation, retinopathy of prematurity, intraventricular haemorrhage and bronchopulmonary dysplasia.

Periventricular haemorrhage and cerebral ischaemia afflict primarily the very low birthweight (VLBW) baby, but they may occur in any neonate, especially those born asphyxiated or with sepsis and trauma.

Further reading

Turnbull Sir AC, Chamberlain GC, eds. *Obstetrics*. Sections 10 and 11. Edinburgh: Churchill Livingstone, 1989.

Related topics of interest

Anatomy of the female pelvis, the fetal skull and the fetal circulation (p. 166)
Rhesus disease (p. 311)

NORMAL LABOUR

Normal labour commences at the onset of painful, regular uterine contractions with progressive dilatation and effacement of the cervix, causing descent and rotation of the fetal head, until full dilatation is reached and contractions become expulsive and, with the aid of maternal effort, effect delivery of the fetus, followed by the placenta and membranes.

Normal labour, for the purposes of obstetric management, assumes a term pregnancy, with a singleton fetus and a vertex presentation, after an uncomplicated pregnancy, labour occurring spontaneously without the need for oxytocic stimulation, with no epidural analgesia.

Labour is divided into three stages: the first stage from the onset of labour to full cervical dilatation; the second stage to delivery of the fetus; the third stage is delivery of the placenta and membranes.

The first stage

Labour is a dynamic process, and the definition of progressive change in the cervix makes diagnosis of the onset of labour difficult, leading to a delay in recognizing abnormal labour and creating uncertainty in implementing management protocols.

This can be overcome by repeating the vaginal examination at set intervals of 1, 2 or 4 hours, and by adopting a more rigid definition of the onset of labour. For example at the National Maternity Hospital in Dublin a woman is deemed to be in labour if she has regular painful contractions and a fully effaced cervix, regardless of the degree of dilatation.

Progress in the first stage of labour is monitored by repeated vaginal examinations and recorded on a partogram. The rate of progress is dependent mainly on dilatation of the cervix. The rate of dilatation is plotted onto a graph or cervicogram, as originally described by Friedman in 1955 and since modified by Philpott in Africa and Studd in the UK.

The second stage

At full dilatation, uterine contractions become expulsive and the mother is stimulated to bear down. With each contraction the presenting vertex descends, allowing for some retraction at the end of each contraction, until the widest diameter of the fetal head (biparietal) reaches the introitus (crowning). Thereafter the mother is asked to pant, and subsequent pushing is controlled by the attendant midwife until delivery is effected. Flexion of the head is encouraged and the perineum is protected until the head is delivered and restitution occurs. Delivery is by gentle downward traction on the head to deliver the anterior shoulder, then an upward movement to sweep the posterior shoulder over the perineum followed by the trunk and limbs. The second stage is complete when the umbilical cord is cut.

The average time for the second stage is 1 hour in primiparous and half an hour in multiparous.

The third stage

Active management of the third stage involves the administration of an oxytocic agent with delivery of the anterior shoulder and prompt clamping and cutting of the umbilical cord.

Thereafter controlled cord traction is applied with a hand on the lower abdomen to prevent displacement of the uterus and the signs of placental separation; a gush of dark placental blood, lengthening of the cord and a decreased resistance to the abdominal hand occur. Gentle traction is continued until placenta and membranes are delivered completely.

The physiological method of delivery of the third stage does not allow for the administration of oxytocic drugs. Instead placental separation is encouraged by placing the baby on the breast and/or by nipple stimulation. When separation occurs delivery of the placenta and membranes is effected as described above.

It has been shown that active management reduces the incidence of post-partum haemorrhage and retained placenta.

Further reading

O'Driscoll K, Meagher, D. *Active Management of Labour*. London: Saunders, 1980.
Studd J. (ed.) *The Management of Labour*. Oxford: Blackwell Scientific Publications, 1985.

Related topics of interest

PERINATAL MORTALITY

Definitions

(WHO ninth and tenth Revision of the International Classification of Diseases, interpretation may differ in each country.)

The perinatal period commences at 22 completed weeks (154 days) of gestation (birth weight equivalent to 500 g), and ends 7 days after birth. In this country 24 completed weeks is used as the starting point, late fetal loss describing the time between 20–23 weeks.

The neonatal period commences at birth and ends 28 days after, (early neonatal period: days 0–6, late neonatal period: days 7–27). The postneonatal period extends from 28 days to 364 completed days after birth.

Perinatal mortality rate (PNMR) is the number of stillbirths, plus deaths in the first week, per 1000 total deliveries.

In this country the PNMR has fallen steadily from around 500 in deprived areas in the 1850s to 32.8 in 1960 to 7.6 in 1993. The main reasons for this decline include improved general health and education of the population, improved maternity and neonatal services, reduced parity and better antenatal screening. Neonatal mortality rates have fallen in a parallel way.

Factors associated with an increased PNM

1. Maternal. >35 years, parity (1 or >4), low socio-economic class, heavy smoking, height < 5ft (152 cm).

2. Bad past obstetric history. Premature labour, APH, LSCS, perinatal deaths.

3. Current pregnancy. APH, diabetes, hypertension, Rhesus isoimmunization, severe anaemia, IUGR, multiple pregnancy, polyhydramnios, oligohydramnios, premature labour, post maturity.

Despite advances, the cause of most stillbirths remains unknown. Consequently, the Confidential Enquiry into Stillbirths and Deaths in Infancy (CESDI) was set up. In addition to data collection it aims to identify ways in which these deaths may be prevented.

**Classification of causes of
perinatal mortality
(extended Wigglesworth)**

- Congenital defect/malformation (e.g. spina bifida, cardiac anomalies, serious biochemical abnormalities e.g. Tay Sach's disease).
- Unexplained antepartum stillbirth (intrauterine anoxia).
- Intrapartum asphyxia, anoxia or trauma.
- Immaturity (respiratory distress syndrome [RDS], intraventricular haemorrhage [IVH]).
- Infection (e.g. Group B streptococci, rubella, parvovirus, syphilis).
- Other specific causes (fetal e.g. hydrops fetalis, neonatal e.g. pulmonary hypoplasia).
- Accident + trauma.
- Sudden infant death syndrome.

The main contribution to the decling perinatal and neonatal mortality during the last 10 years has been a 50% reduction in deaths from congenital malformation, associated with improved antenatal screening and survival following treatment. An ultrasound scan should be offered to all pregnant women; it will detect up to 70% of gross abnormalities and all multiple pregnancies. The correct dating of a pregnancy may reduce the induction rates, but ultrasound only alters perinatal mortality by identifying abnormal fetuses that are subsequently aborted. Rates may be reduced further by patient education (promotion of folic acid, avoidance of drugs in early pregnancy) and advances in screening (nuchal cord thickness, triple test etc). Diabetic control should be optimized prior to pregnancy, to reduce the rates of abnormalities linked to this disease. In the future pre-implantation diagnosis may decrease deaths from hereditary disease.

A decline in antepartum stillbirth has contributed most to the overall decline in stillbirth rates, but unexplained stillbirths remain the largest problem. The fourth CESDI report concentrated on intrapartum related deaths (1994–1995), over two thirds of all cases were considered to be associated with suboptimal care, 70% of which occurred during labour. Recommendations to reduce this include improved use and interpretation of CTGs and fetal blood sampling and avoidance of delay in operating once a compromised fetus has been identified. Training in neonatal resuscitation and enhanced communication (both written records and handovers) are needed.

Death from prematurity and its consequences is the second commonest cause of deaths. There have been no significant change in these rates since 1992, attributable to an increase in the registration of these births, possibly as a result of the early delivery of babies at risk of stillbirth. Corticosteroids should be given to women in premature labour under 36 weeks, to decrease the incidence of RDS and IVH. Tocolytics for 48 hours may delay delivery to allow the steroids to work, and to enable transport of the woman to a tertiary care centre with neonatal facilities. Cervical cerclage will decrease premature deliveries in women who have previously had cervical incompetence.

Mortality due to infections is decreasing slowly, but it still accounts for significant perinatal and neonatal deaths. Antenatal screening for syphilis and rubella should continue, and high risk populations should be screened for HIV and hepatitis. Women who are known to have group B streptococcus isolated from the genital tract or urine, should be given intravenous antibiotics whilst in labour. Prompt treatment of suspected intrauterine infection is essential.

Further reading

Confidential Enquiry into Stillbirths and Deaths in Infancy. 4th Annual Report, 1 January–31 December 1995. Maternal and Child Health Research Consortium, London, 1997.

Effective procedures in maternity care suitable for audit. RCOG Clinical Audit Unit, RCOG London, 1997.

Neale R. Intrapartum Stillbirths and Deaths in Infancy: The First CESDI report. *Progress in Obstetrics and Gynaecology*, **12:** 193–211.

Related topics of interest

Infection in pregnancy (p. 232)
Monitoring in labour (p. 245)
Preconceptual assessment (p. 274)
Premature labour (p. 276)
Prenatal diagnosis (p. 281)

PHYSIOLOGY OF PREGNANCY

In a normal, singleton pregnancy the physiological changes of pregnancy are positive and adapt to meet fetal demands in a favourable way, are reversible, and cause no permanent damage to the mother. Physiology may turn into pathophysiology and first pregnancies are less physiological than subsequent ones. Physiological changes in pregnancy begin soon after conception.

General

Average weight gain in pregnancy is 12.5 kg, with the rate of gain being fairly constant throughout a pregnancy. There is a positive correlation between maternal weight gain and birthweight. The main factor in weight gain is water; of the order of 8.5 kg. The fetal component (everything contained within the gravid uterus) at term is responsible for almost 5 kg (40%) of the weight gained. Joint laxity and postural change, secondary to the alteration in the axis and position of the maternal centre of gravity, are very common, and lead to an altered gait at term and many of the aches and pains in pregnancy, including hip and back pain. Oedema is ubiquitous and may lead to tracheal and intubation problems. The exact calorific requirements of a pregnancy are in dispute, but are of the order of 50–100 kcal/day up to 36 weeks and 200–300 kcal/day thereafter. There is an increased blood flow to the skin, sweat and sebaceous glands are more active and there may be increased body and facial hair. The subcutaneous tissue is thickened, leading to the coarsened facial features seen in many at term, and pigmentation of the face (chloasma or 'mask of pregnancy'), nipples, umbilicus, vulva and scars may increase. Striae gravidarum, especially of the abdominal wall, buttocks and thighs, occurs secondary to the rapid and excessive skin stretching in these areas. Breast development is accentuated after 8 weeks and is mainly the result of glandular hyperplasia and hypertrophy and fat deposition. Colostrum may be expressed from the second trimester. The osmoregulatory system for diuresis and thirst is set 6–8 mosmol/kg lower. Aldosterone is raised, being eight- to tenfold greater at 36 weeks than in the non-pregnant state. The increase in progesterone and glomerular filtration rate (GFR) causes sodium loss and potassium retention, but the increase in plasma renin substrate resulting from increased oestrogen and progesterone activates the renin-angiotensin-aldosterone cascade, thereby balancing the sodium loss and volume depletion effects of progesterone. It is this renal retention of sodium that causes the water retention noted above. Angiotensin is raised twofold, but its pressor effects are checked by increased synthesis of the vasodilatory prostaglandins PGE2 and prostacyclin, PGI2.

Cardiovascular

Blood volume increases by between 1250 and 1500 ml, reaching a zenith at 34–36 weeks. This is caused more by an increase in plasma volume than by an expansion in red cell mass, and hence a physiological haemodilutional anaemia occurs; the WHO lower level of normal is 11.0 g/dl. Mean cell volume (MCV) is steady or rises from 82–84 fl to 86–100 fl by term. It is greater if haematinics are used. The packed cell volume (PCV) declines correspondingly. Stroke volume rises by 10% and pulse rate by 15/min. Cardiac output is increased by 1.5 l/min to 6.5–7.0 l/min at 10 weeks and remains so until term. It increases by about 30% to 8 l/min in the first stage of labour and by 50% to 9 l/min in the second stage. The arterial blood pressure does not rise in parallel with the increase in cardiac output, primarily because of the drop in hormonally mediated peripheral vascular resistance and vessel dilatation. It normally falls on average by 5 mmHg systolic and 15 mmHg diastolic prior to 20 weeks, rising to prepregnancy levels at term. The effect of the gravid uterus on the aorta and the inferior vena cava may drastically alter maternal haemodynamics, e.g. supine hypotension and syncope, so it is important to measure blood pressure with a correctly sized cuff on a relaxed patient sitting, or semirecumbent and tilted to the left. The fourth Korotkoff sound should be used. Venous blood pressure is only slightly raised in pregnancy in most parts of the body, but it is significantly raised in the dependent lower limbs. As a consequence of the hyperdynamics of pregnancy many women develop cardiac murmurs. In the absence of symptoms or signs of cardiac compromise they do not warrant investigation.

Respiratory

The thoracic cage is lifted up and the ribs flare, there is an increased AP diameter, an elevation and increased excursion of the diaphragm, except towards term where it reduces, and the heart rotates forward, which needs to be accounted for in a maternal ECG. The respiratory rate does not generally increase, but the tidal volume does by 200 ml and the vital capacity by 100–200 ml. This hyperventilation causes a mild alkalaemia; arterial pH = 7.44. The effect of all of these changes, plus the reduction of the maternal respiratory centre threshold to pCO_2 stimulus (probably due to progesterone) by a rise of 1 mmHg, increases the maternal minute volume to 6 l/min. It also facilitates gas exchange from the fetus to the mother and, in conjunction with the high levels of oestrogen causing increased maternal respiratory centre sensitivity, it makes the mother prone to dyspnoea and dizziness. These physiological changes have a significant affect on anaesthesia during pregnancy.

Renal

See Renal tract in pregnancy.

Gastrointestinal

Appetite may change early, and nausea and vomiting is very common, along with cravings for unusual substances (pica). Salivary excretion is increased and gastric secretion and motility are decreased. Gut transit times are increased, and water retention (whether or not due to haematinics) promotes constipation in conjunction with the physical obstruction from the growing uterus and fetus. Gastro-oesophageal reflux is common owing to increased gastric pressure and loss of tone at the cardia. Cholestasis is physiological and can lead to pruritus, but rarely jaundice. Alkaline phosphatase rises, but it originates mostly from the placenta. Interpreting liver function in pregnancy is difficult. Although hepatic function is relatively unchanged, other changes, such as those seen in the kidneys, may significantly alter maternal drug metabolism. All lipids rise in pregnancy, predominantly cholesterol and triglycerides.

Endocrine

See Diabetes and pregnancy and Thyroid and pregnancy.

Further reading

Davey DA. Normal pregnancy: physiology and antenatal care. In: Whitfield CR, ed. *Dewhurst's Textbook of Obstetrics and Gynaecology for Postgraduates*, 4th edn. Oxford: Blackwell Scientific Publications, 1988; 126–58.

Related topics of interest

Diabetes and pregnancy (p. 196)
Renal tract in pregnancy (p. 305)
Thyroid and pregnancy (p. 314)

POLYHYDRAMNIOS/OLIGOHYDRAMNIOS

The assessment of reduced (*oligohydramnios*) or excessive (*polyhydramnios*) volumes of liquor are clinically highly subjective. The use of USS has enabled a semiquantitative method of fluid volume determination. The largest pocket is identified and measured. Fluid volume is defined as normal when the largest pocket measures >2 cm and <8 cm in its maximal vertical diameter.

Polyhydramnios is therefore defined as a pool depth of greater than 8 cm with a pool depth less than 2 cm (in some reports 1 cm) defined as oligohydramnios.

Aetiology

Polyhydramnios is dealt with elsewhere (see Hydrops fetalis). Oligohydramnios can result from the following:

- Congenital anomalies, e.g. Potter's syndrome.
- PET.
- IUGR and its associated causes.
- PROM.
- Prolonged pregnancy.
- Raised AFP is an association.

Potential problem

The incidence of major lethal anomalies is lowest in patients with normal liquor and increased 17-fold with increased fluid and 32-fold with decreased fluid. Likewise, perinatal mortality is increased sevenfold with polyhydramnios and 40-fold with oligohydramnios. Intervention for oligohydramnios has been shown to improve perinatal survival rates.

Risks associated with polyhydramnios are an unstable lie, cord prolapse, premature labour, PROM, placental abruption and increased risk of PPH. Tapping of fluid in severe cases is possible, but only causes brief respite from symptoms and can be associated with premature labour and introduction of infection into the amniotic cavity. Recently, the use of indomethacin has been advocated to reduce liquor volume by decreasing fetal urine output.

Risks associated with oligohydramnios are IUGR, chronic intrauterine asphyxia and intrauterine death.

The importance of oligohydramnios as a parameter in the biophysical profile has already been established. The reason that fluid is decreased in chronic hypoxia is that fetal blood flow will be diverted away from fetal lungs and kidneys, which are the two main areas of amniotic fluid production.

Management   USS is used to confirm the diagnosis and exclude fetal anomaly. In oligohydramnios the fetus must be viewed as high risk, and regular fetal assessment must be performed and results acted upon.

Polyhydramnios management is dealt with elsewhere.

Further reading

Chamberlain PF, Manning FA, Morrison I *et al.* Ultrasound evaluation of amniotic fluid I and II. *American Journal of Obstetrics and Gynecology*, 1984; **150:** 245–50.

Related topics of interest

POST-PARTUM HAEMORRHAGE

The risk of maternal death from PPH is approximately 1 in 1000 in developing countries (28% of maternal deaths) and 1 in 100 000 in Britain.

Primary post-partum haemorrhage is defined as blood loss from the genital tract in excess of 500 ml within the first 24 hours after delivery of the baby.

Secondary post-partum haemorrhage is defined as excessive bleeding from the genital tract after 24 hours post-partum and until 6 weeks after the birth.

The incidence of primary PPH varies from between 2–11%. It is notoriously difficult to estimate blood loss; a loss of 15% of the blood volume will result in hypotension. PPH may be best defined by a fall in haematocrit or need for transfusion. It is the commonest cause of serious blood loss and accounted for eight deaths in the UK between 1991 and 1993.

Aetiology

1. Uterine atony. This accounts for 90% of PPH. There are a number of factors associated with uterine atony:

- Uterine overdistension.
- Retained products.
- Multiparity impairs uterine contraction.
- Antepartum haemorrhage especially abruptio placentae.
- Prolonged labour.
- LSCS and forceps delivery.
- Previous history of a PPH.

2. Trauma to the genital tract. For example, tears. episiotomy, cervical tears and in the worst extreme uterine rupture.

3. Coagulation disorders. In patients with inherent coagulation disorders such as von Willebrand's disease or ITP, or those with acquired disease, PPH should be predicted. However acute coagulopathies can develop from for example amniotic fluid embolism. Rarely, drugs such as warfarin and nifedipine can result in a predisposition to a PPH.

Management

Initially preventive with active management of the third stage. Mismanagement can result in severe PPH from retained placenta and uterine inversion.

Syntometrine (5 IU syntocinon + 0.5 mg ergometrine) given IM with the delivery of the anterior shoulder, reduces the blood loss in third stage and reduces the risk of PPH by >40%. Ergometrine can reduce the incidence of PPH.

The first step in the treatment of PPH must be resuscitation by obtaining an intravenous access, blood for X-match, setting up a syntocinon infusion. If the cause were felt to be atony and ergometrine had not been given, then 0.5 mg of ergometrine should be administered IV. The bladder should be catheterized.

The abdomen should be palpated; if the uterus is well contracted the likely cause is genital tract trauma. The placenta must be removed if it is retained and if already delivered must be checked for completeness. Uterine inversion must be treated if present by GA and hydrostatic reduction. Inversion can cause profound shock and needs to be reduced as an emergency; a laparotomy may be required.

If bleeding has not stopped then an EUA should be performed to exclude retained products, trauma to the upper vagina, cervix, uterus.

If all is normal and diagnosis is still uterine atony, then 250 µg carboprost ($PGF_{2\alpha}$ analogue) IM can be administered which can be repeated if necessary. This is effective in up to 88% of patients. Direct intra-myometrial injection of prostaglandins is faster and more effective. Gemeprost pessaries inserted into the uterus have also been proven to be successful. The use of boiling hot water as a douche has been used in the past, but care must be taken to avoid burning the patient's perineum and thighs. Tranexamic acid 1g IV has also been used successfully.

Massive obstetric haemorrhage

This is defined as >1000 ml of blood loss. It occurs after 1.3% of deliveries in Britain.

The treatment should be multidisciplinary, with input from both obstetricians and anaesthetists. If medical treatment of uterine atony is unsuccessful then hysterectomy may be necessary. This is particularly good in treating haemorrhage due to persistent atony, a morbidly adherent placenta and for uterine rupture, although repair in this case may be possible. Ligation of the internal iliac artery has been suggested but only appears to be successful in controlling half those patients with PPH secondary to atony. Successful uterine packing has been described in the USA, and a case report used a Sengstaken-Blakemore tube (usually used to control bleeding varices).

Active resuscitation with blood substitutes and blood (initially group O) must be given and careful monitoring of central venous pressure and fluid balance with a urinary catheter must be performed.

Massive blood transfusion has its own side effects, and in severe haemorrhage it may be necessary to transfer the patient to an ITU as there are risks of developing DIC and ARDS, both from shock and through massive blood transfusion.

Secondary PPH

The incidence is between 0.5–1.5%. It is often due to infection of retained products. The products undergo necrosis which can prevent involution of the placental site and result in secondary haemorrhage.

Infection and dehiscence of a LSCS scar, rupture of a vulval haematoma and rarely the development of choriocarcinoma can result in a secondary PPH.

Secondary PPH usually occurs during the second week post-delivery. It can result in severe haemorrhage with the woman arriving in a state of shock.

Treatment should be resuscitation, followed by a coarse of broad-spectrum antibiotics for 24 hours prior to an evacuation if time permits. Evacuation should be performed by an experienced surgeon as the risk of uterine perforation is increased. Curettings must be sent for histological analysis to exclude choriocarcinoma.

It must be remembered that in certain religions blood transfusions are prohibited (Jehovah's Witnesses).

Further reading

Burke G, Duignan NM. Massive obstetric haemorrhage. In: Studd J, ed. *Progress in Obstetrics and Gynaecology*, Vol 9. 1991; **7**: 111–30.

Drife JO. Management of primary post partum haemorrhage. *British Journal of Obstetrics and Gynaecology*, 1997; **104**: 275–7.

McGrath J, Browne ADH. Use of syntometrine in Rotunda Hospital maternity service. *British Medical Journal*, 1962; **2**: 524–5.

Revised guidelines for the management of massive obstetric haemorrhage. Report on confidential enquiries into Maternal Deaths in the United Kingdom in 1988–1990. London: HMSO, Department of Health, 1994: 43–4.

Related topics of interest

PRE-ECLAMPSIA, ECLAMPSIA AND PHAEOCHROMOCYTOMA

In the latest Triennial Report on Confidential Enquiries into Maternal Deaths in the United Kingdom, eclampsia and pre-eclampsia (PET) accounted for 20 deaths, which is a 26% reduction from the 27 deaths recorded in the previous two triennia. There were 11 cases of deaths due to eclampsia. Although the precise pathology is unknown, altered spiral artery function is involved. PET involves all maternal systems, especially the cardiovascular, coagulation, renal, central nervous and hepatic. Five to ten per cent of primigravidae are affected.

Associated factors

1. Maternal

- Primiparity.
- Previous PET.
- Age <20 or >35.
- Short stature.
- Migraine.
- Family history.
- History of hypertension.
- Raynaud's disease.
- Underweight.
- SLE.

2. Fetal

- Multiple pregnancy.
- Hydrops fetalis.
- Hydatidiform mole.

Diagnosis

Diagnosis is generally made after 20 weeks' gestation. PET may be asymptomatic or be associated with definite symptoms such as flashing lights, photophobia, headache, visual field loss, epigastric pain and vomiting. Hypertension is found, defined as a BP >140/90 mmHg. This definition will account for 20% >20 weeks; 1% will have a BP >170/110 mmHg. Proteinuria (>300 mg/24 h is significant) may be present and if so warrants admission. Oedema is generally present. Weight gain of >2 kg/week is significant, as are retinal changes, hyper-reflexia and sustained clonus. IUGR, oligohydramnios and IUFD may be found.

Investigations	• Four-hourly BP, daily urinalysis and weighing.
	• Full blood count to exclude anaemia and thrombocytopenia.
	• Urate and creatinine to assess renal function.
	• AST, total protein and albumin to assess hepatic function.
	• MSU to assess infection, haemoglobinuria and casts.
	• 24 hour urine collection to assess proteinuria.
	• 24 hour urinary VMA for phaeochromocytoma.
	• Fetal assessment, including BPP and estimated fetal weight.

Management

Management is dictated by the severity of the disease and the gestational age. Admission is warranted. Delivery of the fetus and placenta is the ultimate treatment. In early-onset PET the aim is to continue gestation until at the very least fetal viability is assured (>28 weeks).

Treatment

Short-term treatment (BP >170/110 mmHg rechecked at 15 minutes) is with nifedipine, 10 mg s.l., repeated at 30 minutes prn, or hydralazine, 10 mg IM or IV. Nifedipine is associated with headaches and palpitations as it is a vasodilator, whilst hydralazine may produce rapid hypotension. Diazoxide and labetalol may also be used.

Long-term treatment begins with methyldopa, 500 mg p.o. loading, followed by 250–750 mg q.d.s. It may sedate in the first 48 hours. Slow-release nifedipine may be added to this, up to 20 mg q.i.d., and/or labetalol up to 200 mg q.i.d. Following delivery oxprenolol should be used, up to 80 mg q.i.d., for up to 6 weeks.

Delivery

Allowing the pregnancy to continue beyond 36–37 weeks' gestation is not advised in proteinuric pre-eclamptics as the fetus is mature enough for delivery and the disease will inevitably worsen. Delivery may be best performed by IOL or LSCS, depending upon the severity of the disease, gestation, fetal size and presentation and cervical score. Epidural analgesia is safe provided the platelet count is $80–100 \times 10^{12}/l$. A bleeding time may be necessary to confirm normal platelet function. General anaesthesia with intubation can be difficult because of PET-associated laryngeal

Eclampsia

oedema. All severely affected patients should remain in hospital for a week post-natally, until the risk of eclampsia is over.

Eclamptic convulsions occur antenatally (50%) and post-natally (50%), generally within 24 hours of delivery. Treatment includes maintaining the airway and giving 100% oxygen. Intravenous access should be established and the convulsion arrested with IV diazepam in 10 mg boluses. It is now clear from the Collaborative Eclampsia Trial that further anticonvulsant therapy should be in the form of magnesium sulphate, and all obstetric units should have a written set of guidelines or protocols incorporating this drug. General anaesthesia with thiopentone (a potent anticonvulsant) may be required to control severe convulsions. Delivery is expedited, once control is established, in antenatal eclampsia.

HELLP syndrome

HELLP stands for haemolysis, elevated liver enzymes, low platelets. This presents with severe epigastric pain and significant thrombocytopenia, and may result in hepatic rupture, renal failure and profound DIC. The treatment is primarily supportive with FFP, blood and platelet transfusion, analgesia and antihypertensive therapy. Renal dialysis may be necessary. Antenatal cases will require delivery.

Phaeochromocytoma

This is a very rare cause of hypertension, with a fetal mortality of up to 50%. Diagnosis is made on history, examination, elevated urinary VMA, renal USS or MRI. Treatment is with alpha-adrenergic blockade.

Prognosis after PET

Chronic hypertension may follow PET. The recurrence rate is of the order of 5%, and recurrence is associated with an increase in cardiovascular complications in later life.

CLASP

CLASP stands for collaborative low-dose aspirin in pregnancy. This is an international, double-blind, prospective, randomized, multicentre study looking at the effect of low-dose aspirin (60 mg daily), compared with placebo, on the incidence and progression of pre-eclampsia in primigravidae and multigravidae. Previous studies have shown such antiplatelet therapy to be of benefit in selected high-risk primigravidae.

Further reading

Eclampsia Trial Collaborative Group. Which anticonvulsant for women with eclampsia? Evidence from the Collaborative Eclampsia Trial. *Lancet.* 1995; **345:** 1455–63.

Redman CWG. Hypertension in pregnancy. In: Turnbull Sir AC, Chamberlain GC, eds. *Obstetrics.* Edinburgh: Churchill Livingstone, 1989; 515–42.

Related topics of interest

Immunology of pregnancy (p. 225)
Physiology of pregnancy (p. 260)
Report on Confidential Enquiries into Maternal Deaths in the United Kingdom 1991–1993 (p. 309)
Report on the National Confidential Enquiry into Perioperative Deaths (NCEPOD) (p. 122)

PRECONCEPTUAL ASSESSMENT

This involves a thorough assessment of both partners prior to conception, the aim being to identify and if possible modify any risk factors to mother and/or fetus. Genetic counselling may be appropriate to quantify the risks of fetal malformation and to make arrangements for antenatal diagnosis. General advice with regard to achieving the optimum physical condition, especially of the prospective mother, is given, and treatment of pre-existing disease may be modified to prepare for the proposed pregnancy.

Congenital factors

A family history of congenital abnormality or delivery of a child with a congenital anomaly are indications for genetic counselling.

Risks of an affected pregnancy may be quantified, aided where appropriate by chromosome analysis of family members. When the decision is made to embark on a further pregnancy, then antenatal diagnosis in the first trimester can be arranged.

Acquired factors

General measures to improve pregnancy outcome include: advice to improve diet, weight reduction where appropriate, limiting alcohol intake and stopping smoking. Regular gentle exercise may be beneficial, especially in improving abdominal and pelvic muscle tone. A recent publication from the Department of Health suggests the administration of preconceptual folic acid to prevent neural tube defects.

Specific measures depend on the nature of any underlying disease process.

A thorough drug history is taken and prescriptions altered where possible, bearing in mind that this must not jeopardize the mother's health, e.g. patients with epilepsy may tolerate a reduced dose of anticonvulsants.

Therapy of chronic conditions may be intensified to achieve a prolonged remission during pregnancy, e.g. aggressive use of steroids prior to pregnancy in women with inflammatory bowel disease.

Cardiac and renal conditions must be stable and judged to be able to withstand the physiological changes of pregnancy.

Diabetic control must be optimized, within narrow limits, as this is thought to reduce the incidence of congenital anomalies.

Obstetric factors   A thorough obstetric history is an essential requirement and case notes should be available.

Planning antenatal and intrapartum care may benefit the couple psychologically, with measures such as insertion of cervical sutures and elective Caesarean section discussed.

Conclusion   Preconceptual assessment is designed to inform prospective parents as to the risk of congenital anomaly in their baby and to the risk to the mother's health in light of her previous medical and obstetric history. When the decision to proceed is made then management is aimed at promoting the optimal physical and mental condition for a successful pregnancy and delivery.

Further reading

Chamberlain GC. Prepregnancy care. In: Turnbull Sir AC, Chamberlain GC, eds. *Obstetrics*. Edinburgh: Churchill Livingstone, 1989: 207–17.

Related topics of interest

Abortion, spontaneous/recurrent (p. 7)
Hydrops fetalis (p. 223)
Prenatal diagnosis (p. 281)

PREMATURE LABOUR

Defined as the occurrence of regular uterine contractions productive of cervical change prior to 37 completed weeks of gestation from the first day of the last menstrual period. The incidence in developed countries varies between 5 and 10%, but 70–80% of perinatal deaths occur in preterm infants..

Associated factors

1. *Maternal.* Primigravidae, aged <15 or >35, pregnancy weight <50 kg, non caucasion and smoking.

2. *Socio-economic factors.* Lower social class, a heavy or stressful work load, suboptimal antenatal care and single women.

3. *Past reproductive history.* Previous preterm labour (35% recurrence risk, 70% if two or more) second trimester abortions, stillbirths, uterine abnormalities (congenital, fibroids, trauma) and previous bleeding in pregnancy.

4. *Present pregnancy.* Uterine distension, APH, fetal congenital anomalies, maternal illness, retained IUCD, PROM precedes premature labour in 33% of cases.

5. *Genital tract infections. Neisseria gonorrhoea,* group B streptococcus, *Listeria,* bacterial vaginosis, *Chlamydia trachomatis*, mycoplasma, and viral infections (herpes, CMV, rubella, chicken pox). History of PID, IUCD and multiple sexual partners are also important.

6. *Infection.* There is an increased risk of infection with preterm labour – clinically, bacteriologically and histologically in mother and neonate. Bacteria are recovered from 72% of women with chorioamnionitis. 25% of preterm deliveries are attributable to histopathological evidence of chorioamnionitis.
   Raised C-reactive protein (an acute phase reactant, hepatic in origin, released in response to general mediators of tissue inflammation) has been suggested as a marker. Sensitivity 67–88% and specificity of

68–100% for chorioamnionitis in pre-labour premature rupture of the membranes (PPROM).

7. PPROM. Occurs in 2–3% of pregnancies and one-third of preterm deliveries. When they rupture at 28 weeks, 25% of women remain undelivered after 1 week. Bacterial colonization has been found in 41% of neonates following PPROM (compared to 28% at term).

Prediction of preterm labour

Risk scoring has a low positive predictive value and poor reproducibility.

Cervical assessment – a study from France, prior to 37 weeks, showed early cervical ripening in 30%. If internal os is dilated, there is a four-fold increase in risk of preterm delivery. However these results have not been reproduced.

Transvaginal ultrasound of cervical lengths has been explored, but sensitivity and positive predictive value are too low to justify it as a screening tool.

Fetal fibronectin may be found in amniotic fluid, placental tissue and the extracellular space of the decidua basalis. It is a glycoprotein that may be released into the endocervix or vagina secondary to mechanical or inflammatory mediated damage to the placenta and membranes. Despite papers showing positive predictive values of 77–83%, its presence only generates moderate improvement in the probabilities of having a preterm delivery within 1 week of detection between 34–37 weeks. Therefore, there is currently nothing to indicate its use as a screening test in low risk population.

Diagnosis

Diagnosis is often difficult, but evidence of cervical change must be present. Cervical dilatation of at least 2 cm or 80% effaced. Usually a contraction frequency of at least 4 in 20 minutes.

Management

It is important to look for a cause. Inhibition of labour beyond 34 weeks is not warranted. Premature rupture of the membranes is not a contraindication to delaying labour.

Corticosteroids are administered to promote pulmonary maturation prior to 36 weeks with the aim of delaying delivery for 48 hours. They also decrease the incidence of intraventricular haemorrhage.

The few absolute contraindications to tocolysis include fetal death, fetal congenital anomaly incompatible with life, and chorioamnionitis. Relative contraindications are maternal conditions necessitating delivery such as pre-eclampsia, cardiac disease (may precipitate heart failure) and multiple pregnancy. Care should be taken in diabetes as corticosteroids may increase the insulin requirement.

Tocolytic agents

These should be used only to reduce delivery rates for 48 hours to allow corticosteroids to act, or appropriate *in utero* transfer to be made.

1. Beta-adrenergic agonists. Smooth muscle relaxants via β_2 receptors. The efficacy is limited by its β_1 CVS side effects.

β_2 selective drugs are salbutamol and ritodrine. They may be successful in delaying delivery for more than 7 days. There is no evidence to support oral maintenance therapy.

Maternal side effects are palpitations, pulmonary oedema, nausea and vomiting, diabetogenic symptoms, tremor, headache and restlessness. Rarely death can occur due to fluid overload resulting in pulmonary oedema, cardiac arrhythmias and myocardial ischaemia. It is therefore essential to monitor blood for U&Es, sugar and to have an ECG in progress.

Fetal side effects are tachycardia and hyperglycaemia.

2. Magnesium sulphate. Inhibits myometrial contractility as it competes with calcium for entry into the cell at depolarization. Mg levels need to be 4–7 mmol/l to inhibit contractility.

Careful blood level monitoring is important. Its success is reported to be similar to that of β-adrenergic agonists. Side effects are peripheral vasodilatation, lethargy, fall in maternal temperature. High levels can depress respiration and cause cardiac arrest.

Contraindicated in myasthenia gravis and care in renal impairment.

3. Prostaglandin synthetase inhibitors. Indomethacin is used as $PGF_{2\alpha}$ and PGE_2 are thought to be involved in the final pathway in smooth muscle contraction. It can be administered orally or rectally.

Fetal side effects are renal dysfunction resulting in oligohydramnios, premature closure of ductus arteriosus, intracranial haemorrhage and necrotising enterocolitis. They have been reported to be associated with PPH.

4. Calcium channel blockers. These inhibit the influx of calcium ions through channels in the cell membrane, e.g. nifedipine. They may cause reduced uterine blood flow, but have been shown to be as effective as ritodrine with fewer side effects.

5. Miscellaneous. Ethanol acts both centrally by suppressing the release of ADH and oxytocin from the posterior pituitary.

Diazoxide has a uterine relaxant effect.

Potassium channel openers are potent smooth muscle relaxants and are currently under investigation.

Nitric oxide may inhibit uterine activity (clearly demonstrated in animal models) and nitric oxide compounds may prolong pregnancy after fetal surgery and spontaneous preterm labour.

The role of prophylactic antibiotics is currently under investigation by the ORACLE trial using augmentin and/or erythromycin in women in either preterm labour or with PPROM. However if β-haemolytic streptococcus is present, treatment during labour with 1 g ampicillin IV every 6 hours reduces the incidence of neonatal infection.

Discussion

The use of glucocorticoids prior to 36 weeks is now widely accepted in promoting pulmonary maturation.

Preterm labour may progress despite maximal therapy. It is essential that delivery occurs in a hospital equipped to care for the premature infant.

Survival of infants weighing >1000 g (28 weeks) is approximately 90%.

There is no evidence that Caesarean section for preterm vertex infants improves outcome.

No controlled studies exist for breech delivery of the preterm infant, but several retrospective reports suggest that Caesarean section for footling breech and for infants weighing between 800–1500 g improve the outcome.

Further reading

β-agonists for the care of women in preterm labour. RCOG Guidelines No.1a, 1997.

Alger LS, Crenshaw MC. Preterm labour and delivery of the preterm infant. In: Turnbull Sir AC, Chamberlain GC, eds. *Obstetrics*. Edinburgh: Churchill Livingstone, **50:** 749–70.

Chein PFW, Khan KS, Ogston S, Owen P. The diagnostic accuracy of cervico-vaginal fetal fibronectin in predicting preterm delivery: an overview. *British Journal of Obstetrics and Gynaecology,* 1997; **104:** 436–44.

Crowley P, Chalmers I, Keirse MJ. The effect of corticosteroid administration before preterm delivery: an overview. *British Journal of Obstetrics and Gynaecology,* **97:** 11–25.

Lamont RF, Fisk N. The role of infection in the pathogenesis of preterm labour. In: Studd J, ed. *Progress in Obstetrics and Gynaecology*, Vol 10. Edinburgh: Churchill Livingstone, 1993; 135–58.

Related topics of interest

PRENATAL DIAGNOSIS

This is a rapidly developing field which is expanding further with the advent of pre-implantation diagnosis. Common conditions like neural tube defects (NTDs) and Down's syndrome are most widely screened for, other conditions like cystic fibrosis, haemoglobinopathies, Duchenne muscular dystrophy and fragile-X syndrome can be detected.

Neural tube defects

Spina bifida, anencephaly, encephalocele. The commonest severe congenital abnormality detected at birth with an incidence of up to 2/1000 in some regions. A positive family history is associated with a greater risk (~2% recurrence if one affected child), 3–4% for women with spina bifida themselves. Recurrence can be drastically reduced by taking supplemental folic acid: 5 mg per day. Biochemical and biophysical screening are used.

Biochemical screening is performed for open spina bifida using the measurement of maternal serum alpha-fetoprotein (AFP). Anencephaly can be detected by USS as well as a raised AFP.

AFP is an alpha-globulin synthesized in the yolk sac and fetal liver. By 17 weeks AFP is present in fetal CSF and serum, in open NTD the AFP leaks into the amniotic fluid and thence into the maternal serum, hence the basis for the test. The optimum gestation for detection of open NTD is between 15–17 weeks gestation. AFP values are expressed as multiples of the median (MoM), a compromise figure of 2.5 MoMs will detect 79% of open spina bifida, whereas only 3% of normal pregnancies will have values this high.

Causes of a high AFP are:

- Open neural tube defects (spina bifida, anencephaly).
- Anterior abdominal wall defects.
- Bleeding in the first trimester.
- Non-caucasion women.
- Intrauterine death, Rhesus haemolytic disease.
- Fetomaternal haemorrhage, e.g. after amniocentesis.
- Potter's syndrome, urethral obstruction.
- Turner's syndrome (cystic hygroma), nuchal pad.

- Oesophageal atresia, duodenal atresia.
- Multiple pregnancy: 5 MoM for twins.

Women who have a high AFP should have a detailed USS to confirm gestation, singleton pregnancy and an anomaly scan to rule out fetal anomaly.

The measurement of amniotic fluid AFP has been suggested in borderline cases, but more importantly the use of acetylcholinesterase band in gel electrophoresis (NTD) or the presence of a pseudocholinesterase band (anterior abdominal wall defects) can be very useful. With the use of this active screening test the birth prevalence of anencephaly and spina bifida has declined by 80% in the last 20 years.

Biophysical (USS) assessment is essential in these cases. The signs are described below:

(a) Anencephaly: Absence of fetal cranial vault.
(b) Spina bifida: Open spina bifida is the most common cause of hydrocephalus in early pregnancy. Other associated stigmata are the so called 'Lemon' sign, referring to the shape of the head, and the 'Banana' sign referring to the shape of the cerebellum. It is also important to visualize the defect, commonly lumbo-sacral. Predicting the outcome of spina bifida can be done using prognostic criteria suggested by Lorber. Obviously closed defects have a better prognosis than open.

Down's syndrome

This is (*Trisomy 21*) the commonest cause of mental retardation. 1.3/1000 births in England and Wales are affected by Down's syndrome. The risk increases with advancing maternal age.

Approximately	1 in 1000	(30)
	1 in 450	(35)
	1 in 250	(36)
	1 in 200	(38)
	1 in 100	(40)
	1 in 50	(43)

Only 35% of Down's births occur to women over 35 years of age. Risks of recurrence are increased especially for 14/21 balanced translocation (10% mother carrier, 2% father carrier). Incidence rates have changed little over recent years, despite advances in screening. Biochemical screening has shown that a low AFP result, 0.4 MoM is suggestive of Down's syndrome.

The risks of Down's syndrome is based on maternal age, weight, past history, gestation and the level of AFP. The *triple test* has increased the ways in which prenatal screening for Down's syndrome can be performed. This involves three maternal parameters, serum AFP, maternal serum unconjugated oestriol (uE_3) and human chorionic gonadotrophin (HCG), the free β unit perhaps being most sensitive. Down's syndrome is associated with a low AFP, a low uE_3 and a high HCG.

By combining these three parameters it is possible to give a relative risk of Down's syndrome for that particular pregnancy. A low AFP alone will detect one-third of cases of Down's syndrome whereas the triple test will detect two-thirds of cases, with a false-positive rate of 5%.

Other placental markers have been investigated including pregnancy associated plasma protein-A (PAPP-A), human placental lactogen, cancer antigen 125, placental alkaline phosphotase, progesterone, Schwangerschaft's protein, maternal thyroid antibodies and neutrophil alkaline phosphatase.

Advances are now being sought for first trimester screening when free β HCG seems to be consistently raised, and PAPP-A levels are reduced. Detection (55–62%) and false positive (5%) rates seem to be similar to those for second trimester screening, but further evaluation is required.

Biophysical assessment using ultrasound has also been useful. Nuchal translucency measurement is highly effective marker at 10–13 weeks gestation, detecting 85% of fetal aneuploides when it is increased above 3 mm. Pathological umbilical Doppler pattern (absent or reversed end diastolic velocity) seen during the first trimester has also been suggested as a screening method.

Ultrasonography is also useful in looking for other soft tissue markers associated with Down's syndrome such as duodenal atresia and cardiac abnormalities.

Edward's syndrome

Trisomy 18; the second commonest autosomal trisomy with a birth incidence of 1 in 7000. The incidence increases with maternal age and it is invariably fatal either during the third trimester (70% demise) or shortly after birth.

25% have open neural tube or ventral wall defects. The others have low levels of MSAFP, uE_3 and total free βhCG.

The use of maternal age, MSAFP and free ßhCG detect 50% with a 1% false positive rate.

Ultrasonographic soft tissue markers should detect 85% of these cases, e.g. exompholus, radial aplasia, congenital heart defects, choroid plexus cysts and head profile abnormalities.

Cystic fibrosis

This autosomal recessive condition affects about 1 in 2000 births in the UK, 1 in 22 people are carriers and most cases occur with no relevant family history.

A mouthwash test can detect 82–92% of carriers allowing couples to be effectively screened. Pre-conceptual or antenatal screening can be offered. Initially the woman is screened, if the result is positive their male partner is tested. If he is positive, amniocentesis or chorionic villus biopsy (CVB) is arranged. DNA analysis by polymerase chain reaction is then performed.

Sickle cell disease

This affects African, Indian, Middle Eastern and Mediterranean people; carrier rates of up to 25% have been reported. Prenatal screening begins with at risk women, by haemoglobin electrophoresis. If they screen positive their partners are checked, and if they also screen positive amniocentesis or CVB is offered.

Thalassemias

Homozygous Å-thalassemia may be suggested by hydrops; it is invariably fatal.

β-thalassemia, affecting people from South East Asia, the Middle East and the Mediterranean, with carrier rates of 1 in 7 can be detected in a similar way to sickle cell disease with haemoglobin electrophoresis as the initial step.

Biophysical screening

When gestation is certain the optimum time to perform an USS is between 19–20 weeks when one can assess structure, placental position, biophysical behaviour and gestation within 10 days. The diagnosis is operator dependent with accurate diagnosis being made in 99% of cases in good centres with a false negative rate of under 1%. Specific abnormalities will now be discussed.

1. Craniospinal abnormalities. These account for over 50% of fetal abnormalities. The commonest reasons for referral are a raised AFP, previous history of defect or suggestion of abnormality on an earlier scan.

The commonest two reasons of open neural tube defects have already been discussed. The remainder are:

- Hydrocephalus: The upper level of normal is 8 mm diameter of the anterior horn of the ventricle.
- IVH/ICH: associated dilatation cerebral ventricles.
- Choroid plexus cysts: Very common (1% of pregnancies), usually decrease in size. Significance is still under debate. Mid-trimester detection of isolated cysts increases the risk of Edward's syndrome but not Down's syndrome. When found in isolation the risk of trisomy is about 1 in 150.
- Encephalocele: Rare constituting only 1% of NTD. Not associated with a raised AFP as are skin covered.
- Posterior fossa: Absence of cerebellum is associated with trisomies.
- Rarities: Holoprosencephaly is the presence of a single centrally placed cerebral ventricle and is associated with midline abnormalities especially face and abdomen.

2. Fetal tumours. The commonest two fetal tumours are a *cystic hygroma* and a *sacrococcygeal teratoma*. The former is usually associated with Turner's syndrome. The finding of this therefore warrants karyotyping and detailed fetal echocardiography. Excision of both are possible post delivery.

3. Gastrointestinal. Obstruction of the bowel above the ileum results in polyhydramnios. Duodenal atresia can be recognized by the presence of a double bubble; one-third of such lesions are associated with Down's syndrome.

Diaphragmatic hernia can be diagnosed as cystic areas within the chest. 33% will die antenatally. Recurrence is common in future pregnancies.

An *omphalocele* is a midline defect through which a peritoneal sac containing liver and varying amounts of small bowel are present. They are within the cord and are therefore easily differentiated from gastroschisis. More severe midline abnormalities may also occur such as *ectopica vesicae* and *ectopica cordis*.

25–30% of all fetuses with an omphalocele will have associated cardiac and chromosomal abnormalities (especially trisomy 18), amniocentesis is therefore indicated. If the omphalocele is an isolated lesion then repair is possible and the outcome good.

Gastroschisis is much less common and can be differentiated from the previous lesion because the umbilical cord insertion is intact. Prognosis is very good.

4. Renal tract. Fetal bladder and a normal amount of amniotic fluid are signs of normality.

Renal agenesis is difficult to diagnose as it is based on absence of renal echoes, no bladder filling and oligohydramnios.

Polycystic kidneys and obstructive uropathy are easily seen and diagnosed. Posterior urethral valves occur almost exclusively in males, are associated with a large dilated bladder and varying degrees of renal tract dilatation. 25% of such cases are associated with chromosomal abnormalities and karyotyping should be performed.

5. Limb problems. All fetal long bones can be measured so diagnosing dwarfism. Talipes can also be diagnosed.

6. Facial. Cleft lip and cleft palate can be diagnosed. Cyclops syndrome can also be easily diagnosed.

7. Cardiac. 8:1000 live births will have a cardiac anomaly. 25% will die, 50% are small and either self correcting or easily correctable. Because of the severe problems that a cardiac lesion can cause if the basic four chamber view is abnormal, then it is wise to seek expert advice.

Invasive procedures

1. Amniocentesis. Commonest procedure performed at the present time. Always performed under USS control with a 22 gauge needle inserted away from the head of the fetus. It is performed at 15–16 weeks gestation as the results of cell culture, AFP and acetylcholinesterase are most accurate.

Early amniocentesis (performed before 14 weeks) may be associated with a higher miscarriage rate and is currently being evaluated in a large prospective Canadian study.

Indications

- Chromosomal anomalies (maternal age >37).
- Fetal sexing in X-linked disorders.
- NTD – raised AFP or acetylcholinesterase.
- Bilirubin (management of rhesus disease).
- Phospholipids (fetal pulmonary maturity).
- Symptomatic relief of acute polyhydramnios.

A 10 ml sample of amniotic fluid is removed, with the result available within 3 weeks. The risk of spontaneous abortion following amniocentesis is <1%. A slight increase in postural deformities (talipes) and respiratory difficulties in the neonate have been reported. Fetal trauma during amniocentesis is very rare. Increased fetal loss rates are found in the presence of raised AFP and when the needle is inserted through the placenta.

2. Chorion villus sampling. This should be performed using a transabdominal approach normally between 10–14 weeks, as the cervical route is associated with greater risk of infection, ruptured membranes and abortion. Although initially popular it is now only used in high risk pregnancies. The spontaneous abortion rate of CVS is about 3–4%, so pregnancies with risks of abnormalities greater than 1:25 should only be offered this test. Limb and facial deformities (particularly fingers and nose) following CVS especially if performed before 10 weeks.

Sufficient material is obtained in 98% of cases with a result available much quicker even within 24 hours. The only potential problem is that false positive chromosomal diagnoses may occur due to abnormalities such as mosaicism being present in the villi but not in the fetus. CVS is most beneficial in patients with genetic histories and a 1:2 or 1:4 recurrence risks i.e. haemaglobinopathies, previous Down's, Duchenne muscular dystrophy, cystic fibrosis, inborn errors of metabolism.

3. *Fetal blood sampling.* Performed under USS control and called cordocentesis when the needle is inserted into the umbilical cord at its attachment to the placenta. Fetal blood can also be obtained by inserting the needle into the fetal heart or the hepatic vein although both methods are rarely used.

Indications

- Haemaglobinopathies.
- Chromosome disorders (after a failed amniocentesis).
- Viral and other infections.
- Transfusion and management of Rhesus disease.
- Immunodeficiences.
- Metabolic disorders.
- Non-immune hydrops.
- Fetal blood gas and acid-base measurements in high risk pregnancies.

In experienced hands fetal loss after cordocentesis is approximately 2%. The major risks are fetal exsanguination, haematoma of the cord and chorioamnionitis.

Fetoscopy is now used very rarely and only when small or subtle lesions of diagnostic importance cannot be adequately assessed by USS. It has a high risk of preterm delivery (10%), fetal loss is associated with >5%, and also has a much higher risk of amnionitis and amniotic fluid leakage.

Preimplantation diagnosis Chromosomal abnormalities and single gene defects account for 1–3% of disease in infancy.

Preimplantation diagnosis provides the possibility of primary prevention of these diseases, like cystic fibrosis and X-linked disorders, without the need for terminating the pregnancy.

Embryos are generated by standard IVF techniques, 3 days after insemination; 1–2 cells are biopsied from the 6–10 cell embryos, up to two of the normal embryos are then replaced. By 1996, 29 infants had been born world-wide with no reported congenital malformations, but further monitoring is obviously essential.

Further reading

Chard T, Macintosh MCM. Biochemical screening for Down's syndrome. In: Studd J, ed. *Progress in Obstetrics and Gynaecology*, Vol 11. Edinburgh: Churchill Livingstone, 1994: 39–52.

Gupta JK, Khan KS, Thornton JG, Lilford RJ. Management of fetal choroid plexus cysts. *British Journal of Obstetrics and Gynaecology,* 1997; **104:** 881–6.

Management of fetal choroid plexus Cysts

Nicolaides KH, Soothill PW. Cordocentesis. In: Studd J, ed. *Progress in Obstetrics and Gynaecology,* Vol 7. 1989; **8:** 123–44.

Pearce JM. The biophysical diagnosis of fetal abnormalities. In: Turnbull Sir AC, Chamberlain GC, eds. *Obstetrics.* Edinburgh: Churchill Livingstone, 1989; **20:** 291–308.

Report of the RCOG Working party on ultrasound screening for fetal abnormalities. RCOG January 1997.

Taylor AS, Braude PR. Pre-implantation diagnosis of genetic disease. In: Studd J, ed. *Progress in Obstetrics and Gynaecology*, Vol 11. Edinburgh: Churchill Livingstone, 1994: 3-22

Thornton JG, Onwude JL. Prenatal diagnosis. In: Studd J, ed. *Progress in Obstetrics and Gynaecology,*Vol 10. Edinburgh: Churchill Livingstone, 1993: 13–31.

Soussis I, Harper JC, Handyside AH, Winston RML. Obstetric outcome of pregnancies resulting from embryos biopsied for pre-implantation diagnosis of inherited disease. *British Journal of Obstetrics and Gynaecology,* 1996; **103:** 784–8.

Wald NJ, Cuckle HS. Biochemical detection of neural tube defects and Down's syndrome. In: Turnbull Sir AC, Chamberlain GC, eds. *Obstetrics.* Edinburgh: Churchill Livingstone, 1989; **19:** 269–90.

Related Topics of Interest

PRESENTATIONS AND POSITIONS

When labour is said to proceed normally there is a cephalic presentation, with the occiput as the denominator, which enters the pelvis in the transverse diameter (usually on the left), then rotates anteriorly on the floor of levator ani to deliver in the occipitoanterior position. The presenting part is said to be that which lies over the internal cervical os, and therefore a face or brow may be the presenting part of a cephalic presentation.

Malpresentation and malposition

Predisposing causes

1. Passenger

- Anatomical abnormalities, e.g. sacrococcygeal tumour or anencephaly.
- Physiological abnormalities, e.g. disorders of fetal muscle tone.
- Multiple pregnancy (too many passengers): malpresentation is common in multiple pregnancy.

2. Passages

- Pelvic anomalies, e.g. android or oranthropoid pelvis.
- Pelvic tumours, e.g. fibroids.
- Uterine abnormalities.

3. Powers

- Incoordinate uterine activity.

Management

Diagnosis of any predisposing cause may be made antenatally, allowing planned management, e.g. by Caesarean section or trial of labour.

Diagnosis in labour is not uncommon, always for malpositions (including an abnormal presenting part in a cephalic presentation) and occasionally for malpresentations such as the undiagnosed breech. Subsequent management in labour depends on the progress of labour, especially descent of the presenting part and degree and rate of cervical dilatation, with the condition of the fetus being of paramount importance in the planning of an operative delivery. Other factors that may influence management include age, parity, obstetric and medical history, gestation and the wishes of the parents.

Abnormalities of a cephalic presentation

Confusion exists in the terminology with face and brow 'presentations' included here as they are related to a cephalic presentation when the vertex is not the presenting part.

1. Occipitoposterior. Persistent occipitoposterior position may be compatible with a normal vaginal delivery. Labour is generally slow and the likelihood of vaginal delivery is increased with the use of intravenous oxytocin. Perineal trauma is common and a generous episiotomy is recommended.

With full dilatation and adequate descent of the head, operative vaginal delivery, with rotational or non-rotational forceps or vacuum extraction, is feasible. The method of delivery is largely determined by the experience of the operator.

2. Deep transverse arrest. This may be overcome by intravenous oxytocin. If conditions are favourable then operative vaginal delivery, either by rotational forceps or by vacuum extraction, may be performed.

3. Brow presenting. Spontaneous vaginal delivery will not occur. If persistent, then Caesarean section is usually required. An experienced operator may elect to apply rotational forceps and vaginal delivery may be effected.

4. Face presenting. Compatible with vaginal delivery in the mentoanterior position. Mentoposterior is rare, and descent in the pelvis is unlikely.

Malpresentations

1. Breech presentation. See Breech.

2. Transverse and oblique lie. There is a danger of prolapsed cord if the membranes rupture. Patients are admitted at or near term for observation as many will convert spontaneously to a cephalic or breech presentation.

In the absence of a known predisposing cause, a stabilizing induction may be attempted. In established labour, a prolapsed cord should be immediately excluded and delivery effected by Caesarean section.

A transverse lie with a shoulder presenting and the back under the lower segment presents particular difficulties, and a classical Caesarean section may be the preferred approach.

3. Compound presentation. This is most commonly a limb beside the fetal head and is liable to correct spontaneously. Delivery may be accompanied by significant perineal trauma. A rare but potentially lethal variation is locked twins, for which emergency Caesarean section is performed.

Further reading

Clinch J. Abnormal fetal presentations and positions. In: Turnbull Sir AC, Chamberlain GC, eds. *Obstetrics*. Edinburgh: Churchill Livingstone, 1989: 793–812.

Related topics of interest

Anatomy of the female pelvis, the fetal skull and the fetal circulation (p. 166)
Breech (p. 175)
Caesarean section (p. 179)
Episiotomy (p. 211)
Forceps and ventouse (p. 215)
Monitoring in labour (p. 245)
Multiple pregnancy (p. 248)
Normal labour (p. 255)

PRETERM RUPTURE OF THE MEMBRANES (PROM)

Defined as rupture of the fetal membranes before 37 completed weeks of pregnancy. It occurs in 2–3% of pregnancies but accounts for nearly 50% of preterm deliveries and 10% of perinatal mortality. Therefore many of the conditions associated with premature labour are also associated with PROM. Uterine contractions are not necessarily present with PROM.

Aetiology

May occasionally occur secondary to an aggressive external factor, e.g. amniocentesis. It is usually due to the lack of resistance of the fetal membranes to the intra-amniotic pressure.

Decrease in collagen content has been suggested, with evidence from samples taken at term and when PROM occurs in association with uterine distension. Coital activity and vaginal examinations have been implicated. *E. coli*, bacteroides and Group B haemolytic streptococci are associated with PROM. The bacterial growth is associated with a rise in vaginal pH which weakens the cervical mucus and permits dissolution of the membranes, especially as bacteria generate phospholipase A_2, which can stimulate cervical effacement via stimulation of prostaglandins.

Diagnosis

This can be very difficult. The history is usually classical in that a sudden gush of fluid is followed by a constant trickle unrelated to micturition.

Examination is with a sterile speculum. Visualization of liquor amnii coming from the cervix is obvious; pooling in the posterior fornix is helpful. Presence of meconium and/or vernix will differentiate it from urine or vaginal discharge.

If doubt persists, the pH can be tested as liquor amnii is >7.1. The presence of protein is also diagnostic (rarely found in urine). Liquor amnii will cause a ferning on a glass slide. Nitrazine sticks turn dark blue in higher pH, but false positives can occur in the presence of blood, semen and infections.

Management

Management is dependent on gestation. It precedes about 60% of singleton spontaneous preterm births.

>36 weeks gestation then delivery is the best option. This will occur spontaneously in >80% within 24 and 90% within 48 hours. A significantly higher proportion of nulliparous women deliver spontaneously if they are allowed to wait up to 72 hours. If repeated digital examinations are avoided, there is no increase in infections in the delayed group. If the patient is multiparous, there is no advantage in delaying; therefore induction the following morning is the best course of action.

Prostaglandins can be used safely, and may improve the Bishop score prior to syntocinon, especially in nulliparous women.

32–36 weeks gestation – ensure pulmonary maturity before deciding on delivery.

<32 weeks gestation – prolong gestation in the absence of infection or fetal distress.

<28 weeks gestation – associated with >60% survival, mean latency time between PROM and labour is 4 weeks.

Monitoring of infection using serial WCC, ESR and C-reactive protein have all been used but are non-specific. The regular monitoring of the patient's temperature is a better indication of infection.

The necessity for hospitalization is important for the first 10 days following membrane rupture in early gestation, but after 32 weeks some patients can be managed at home. Successful outpatient management of PROM has been reported.

The risks of prematurity and infection is a delicate balance and is dependent on gestation. The risks of prematurity predominates up to 34 weeks, as after this the perinatal outcome differs little from that at term.

Should infection occur, then delivery should be expedited and intravenous antibiotic cover provided. Prophylactic antibiotics have as yet not been shown to be effective, although the ORACLE trial is currently ongoing.

The use of corticosteroids to stimulate lung maturity following PROM and prior to fetal lung maturity has been shown to be beneficial as a 48 hour course when the gestation is between 28 and 34 weeks and outweighs the risks of sepsis. The use of tocolytics is debatable, although as a postponement of labour in order to facilitate *in utero* transfer following early PROM or to gain 48 hours has some merit. Corticosteroids also decrease the risk of intraventricular haemorrhage. They may increase the WCC within 24 hours, but it should then fall. Elevated levels should raise the suspicion of infection.

Following PROM there is potential for developing pulmonary hypoplasia, positional foot deformities and congenital dislocation of the hip due to development of oligohydramnios. Cord prolapse can occur at the time of the original PROM or when uterine action commences. Fetal distress is also more common due to cord compression, secondary to the oligohydramnios. LSCS is indicated for breech delivery when the estimated weight is between 800–1500 g. If labour has not occurred spontaneously then augmentation should be performed at 37 weeks, although after 34 weeks the neonatal mortality is sufficiently low that the risk of cord prolapse and infection assume greater importance.

Further reading

O'Herlihy C, Turner M. Prelabour spontaneous rupture of the membranes. In: Studd JWW, ed. *Progress in Obstetrics and Gynaecology,* Vol 9. Edinburgh: Churchill Livingstone, 1991; **6:** 99–110.

Related topics of interest

PROLONGED PREGNANCY

The International Federation of Gynecology and Obstetrics (FIGO) quotes World Health Organization (WHO) criteria to define prolonged pregnancy as a 'pregnancy lasting 42 completed weeks or more (294 days or more)'. Prolonged pregnancy is not synonymous with post-maturity, which is a clinical syndrome with the fetus manifesting signs of intrauterine growth retardation. The frequency of prolonged pregnancy is of the order of 10% when dates are certain, and 15% when dates are uncertain.

Diagnosis

Find the exact age of the fetus – by LMP or US (the earlier, the more accurate), quickening, fetal heart sounds, uterine size.

Aetiology

The causes are many including seasonal variation (more common in summer), improved nutrition and living standards, past obstetric history, hereditary and racial factors and hormonal influences. Placental ageing as an aetiological factor has probably been disproved, at electron microscopic levels.

Maternal implications

The main worry is one of maternal anxiety with respect to the estimated date of delivery (EDD) and the actual delivery date. The temptation to induce labour electively needs to be resisted, as it is well shown that Caesarean section rates rise disproportionately in this group when they are induced with a low Bishop score. Appropriate counselling at booking as to the variable lengths of a pregnancy may well allay such anxiety.

Fetal and neonatal implications

This is best expressed in terms of perinatal mortality rate (PNMR). In the past it was believed that a prolonged pregnancy had a significantly higher PNMR than that of a 'normal' gestation pregnancy, i.e. 38–42 weeks inclusive. The figures are still contradictory to a certain extent: figures from Dublin show an almost twofold doubling of the PNMR from 5.0 per 1000 at 37–42 weeks to 9.4 per 1000 after 42 weeks, whereas Bergsjo's study in four Nordic countries showed the PNMR at 42–43 weeks to be equal to that of weeks 41 and 40, and less than that for weeks 37–39. In unscreened populations congenital malformations may be 50% higher in prolonged pregnancies, with up to an eightfold increase in anencephaly, a condition well known to be asssociated with a failure of spontaneous onset of labour. In a screened population, where the pregnancy was uncomplicated, no such differences were observed in a 2-year follow-up. Fetuses in a prolonged pregnancy have greater degrees of ossification and a quarter of them will weigh more than 4000 g.

Management

Elective induction at 42 weeks does not improve neonatal outcome, and indeed the outcome may be worse because of the morbidity and mortality of induction of labour in the face of an uncompromised fetus and an unripe cervix. However, the cervix may remain unfavourable despite accurate dating and an increase in gestation to beyond 42 weeks. It is probably wisest to delay intervention unless it is clinically indicated, allow labour to start naturally, and maintain a close watching brief on the mother and the fetus until spontaneous labour intervenes. Prostaglandin pessaries may aid cervical ripening, and may result in labour.

Intrapartum

Meconium may be more prevalent, but this may be a reflection more of dominant vagal tone (vagal tone dominance increases with gestation) than of true fetal distress. Oligohydramnios can be associated with prolonged pregnancy, and if so should also be taken seriously. These factors notwithstanding, in the uncomplicated singleton prolonged pregnancy there is no documented increase in the incidence of fetal distress in labour. In 25% of prolonged pregnancies the fetus weighs more than 4000 g so anticipation of shoulder dystocia becomes important.

Further reading

Bergsjo P. Post-term pregnancy. In: Studd J, ed. *Progress in Obstetrics and Gynaecology*, Vol. 5. Edinburgh: Churchill Livingstone, 1985; 121–33.
Dooley M M, Studd J. Prolonged pregnancy. In: Turnbull Sir AC, Chamberlain GC, eds. *Obstetrics*. Edinburgh: Churchill Livingstone, 1989; 771–81.

Related topics of interest

PUERPERAL PSYCHOSIS

Depressive feelings are common in the puerperium, with up to 24% of women complaining of depressive symptoms. Frank psychosis is much rarer, having a prevalence of 1–2%.

Symptoms

The commonest complaint is of a persistent lowering of mood. Other symptoms include:

- Difficulty in sleeping (not related to a wakeful infant).
- Feeling sad or tearful.
- Excessive worry about herself or her baby.
- Feelings of rejection toward the baby.
- Lack of self-esteem as a mother.
- Marital problems, including a loss of interest in sexual relations.

Aetiological factors

These are multifactorial. Factors include:

- Depressive feelings during pregnancy.
- Age greater than 30 years.
- History of a mood disorder.
- Premenstrual syndrome, especially premenstrual depression.
- Continuation of breast feeding beyond 3 months.
- Lack of support from partner or parents.
- Stressful events during pregnancy or delivery.

Management

An increased awareness of the high incidence of depressive symptoms and of the possible aetiological factors involved should lead to earlier identification of mothers at risk of progressing to a frank puerperal psychosis.

High-risk patients may benefit from increased social support, beginning in the antenatal period.

Early use of antidepressant drugs may be beneficial; breast feeding may continue if the baby is monitored for drowsiness.

Severe cases require hospital admission, preferably to a suitable mother and baby unit. Treatment is with antipsychotic drugs and electroconvulsive therapy.

Conclusions

Depression is common in the puerperium. Frank psychosis is rarer but may have tragic consequences of suicide or infanticide. Untreated patients may have a prolonged illness continuing into a subsequent pregnancy.

Early recognition and prompt action will benefit these patients and may prevent serious sequelae.

Further reading

Dennerstein L. Postnatal depression. In: Tsakok, Liauw, Yu, eds. *Proceedings of the First International Scientific Meeting of the Royal College of Obstetricians and Gynaecologists*. Singapore: World Scientific, 1992: 203–10.

Related topic of interest

Puerperium and breast feeding (p. 302)

PUERPERAL SEPSIS

Puerperal sepsis was a major cause of maternal mortality until the introduction of basic hygienic practice on the labour ward (after the observations of Semmelweis in the 1840s), coupled with the introduction of antibiotics in the middle of the twentieth century.

Pathology

Causative organisms may be exogenous or endogenous to the lower gastrointestinal tract or more rarely the vagina.

Infective organisms ascend via the lower genital tract under the favourable conditions after delivery and colonize the uterine cavity.

Infection is established and spreads directly through the pelvis and via the bloodstream to cause pelvic sepsis with abscess formation, septic thrombosis of pelvic veins and septicaemia. The end result is septic shock, which carries a high mortality.

Clinical features

Predisposing factors include:

- Prolonged ruptured membranes.
- Prolonged labour with repeated vaginal examinations.
- Operative delivery or other intervention such as internal fetal monitoring or manual rotation.
- Episiotomy or other perineal trauma.
- Retained products of conception or intrauterine blood clot.
- History of pelvic sepsis.

Resistance to infection is lowered by malnutrition, exhaustion, anaemia or intercurrent disease.

Patients are usually febrile with pelvic discomfort and an offensive lochia, which may be increased in amount and associated with an increased blood loss.

Established infection in the pelvis may be very painful. Abscess formation is associated with a swinging pyrexia and signs of shock may supervene.

Management

Diagnosis is on clinical grounds, confirmed by appropriate bacteriological investigation. Treatment should be promptly instituted whilst awaiting antibiotic sensitivities. It is important to cover the more virulent organisms such as the beta-haemolytic streptococci and anaerobic bacteria. The decision to change antibiotic therapy is taken on clinical grounds. It is important to remember rare but potentially fatal pathogens such as *Clostridium welchii* in situations where there is no clinical response to a broad-spectrum antibiotic combination.

Surgical treatment options should always be considered, such as evacuation of the uterus or drainage of perineal or pelvic abscesses.

Conclusion

Puerperal sepsis presents less of a threat to the patient with modern treatment regimens. Prompt diagnosis and treatment, with consideration of antibiotic prophylaxis in high-risk situations, is necessary to keep mortality and morbidity to a minimum.

Further reading

Hurley Dame R. Fever and infectious diseases. In: De Swiet M, ed. *Medical Disorders in Obstetric Practice,* Vol. 2. Oxford: Blackwell Scientific Publications, 1989: 775–96.

Related topics of interest

PUERPERIUM AND BREASTFEEDING

The puerperium

The puerperium is defined as that time after completion of the third stage of labour until such time as the changes of pregnancy revert to the non-pregnant state. This time is traditionally taken as 6 weeks.

Puerperial changes

1. Structural. Uterine involution, cessation of the lochia, return of abdominal muscular tone, fading of striae gravidarum, return of normal renal tract dimensions, tone and bladder volume, loss of vaginal distensibility and return of normal elasticity and capacity (may be delayed by breast feeding).

2. Hormonal. Falling levels of sex steroids and prolactin (unless breastfeeding), return of ovarian function (may be delayed by breastfeeding) secondary to cyclical gonadotrophin release from the pituitary, falling thyroid hormones, a short-lived rise then a fall of urinary 17–ketosteroids, declining plasma cortisol, testosterone, androstenedione, renin, angiotensin II and aldosterone, and a loss of the relative insulin resistance.

3. Physiological. Loss of the average 12.5 kg weight gain of pregnancy, consisting of water loss and products of conception (5 kg) and then a slower loss of 4.25 kg until by 10 weeks post-natally the gravida is 2.25 kg heavier than in the non-pregnant state. An immediate rise then a 4-day fall in the haematocrit and haemoglobin is followed by a steady rise, a fall in plasma volume and leucocyte count and fibrinogen levels, a rise in plasma proteins and osmolality and platelets. The physiological hypercoagulable state of pregnancy lasts for about 7 weeks, which has implications for the duration of thromboembolic treatment. There is a slow fall in cardiac output and circulating blood volume. Blood pressure may remain elevated for a week.

4. Psychological. Education is the key to the psychosocial changes that the new mother (and father) have to face. The loss of an income, the demands and fatigue associated with a dependent baby, return of sexuality and libido, the need for contraception can all be adjusted to with appropriate education and forethought. At least 15% of all new mothers undergo a clinical post-natal depressive illness (over and above the so-called 'third-day blues') and this needs to be appreciated by obstetricians, midwives, health visitors, general practitioners, partners and families of new mothers. Contributing factors will include a relevant past psychiatric or obstetric history (e.g. previous depression, traumatic termination of pregnancy), poor socioeconomic circumstances, a difficult pregnancy, labour and delivery, preterm delivery with a baby in special care, an abnormal baby, stillbirth or intrauterine fetal death. One in 500 to 1000 women will have a puerperal psychosis.

Breastfeeding

The glanduar breast tissue is derived from ectoderm and radiates out from the nipple in 15–20 ducts that lead to ductules and then to secretory alveolar cells. Each alveolus is surrounded by oxytocin-sensitive, contractile, myoepithelial cells, and each duct and ductule is lined by longitudinal contractile cells, resulting in milk release at the nipple under the stimulus of the milk let-down reflex. The milk let-down reflex is mediated by oxytocin (an octapeptide manufactured and released from the supraoptic and paraventricular nuclei of the hypothalamus), which binds to the myoepithelial alveolar cells and longitudinal contractile duct cells. The milk let-down reflex acts synergistically with the prolactin neuroendocrine reflex, and both are required for successful lactation. Following pubertal breast development, the breast shows significant hyperplasia and hypertrophy in pregnancy under the influence of oestrogen, growth hormone, glucocorticoids, progesterone, prolactin, human placental lactogen and prednisolone. Prolactin, the main hormone in lactation, is manufactured by lactotrophs in the anterior pituitary. Its release is augmented by a neuroendocrine reflex initiated by nipple stimulus, e.g. suckling. Such a stimulus blocks release of prolactin inhibitory factors (PIFs), e.g. dopamine, from the hypothalamus and stimulates release of prolactin-releasing factors (PRFs), e.g. thyroid-releasing hormone (TRH). Prolactin binds to receptors on the alveolus and acts at multiple sites to stimulate synthesis of milk constituents. The initial early milk, or colostrum, has high concentrations of proteins, including immunoglobulins. Milk contains all of the constituents necessary for at least the first 6 months of the baby's life. The average daily volume of milk released is of the order of 800–1200 ml and a lactating mother requires a calorific intake of 2000–3000 kcal/day to maintain it. Lactation is associated with amenorrhoea, suppression of ovulation and is contraceptive, with between 1 and 10% of women conceiving whilst breast feeding.

Further reading

Dennis J, Howie P, Charles D, Larsen B, Bonnar J, Forrest, G. Normal puerperium and abnormal puerperium. In: Turnbull Sir AC, Chamberlain GC, eds. *Obstetrics, Sections 8 and 9.* Edinburgh: Churchill Livingstone, 198; 891--954.

Kumar R. Pregnancy, childbirth and mental illness. In: Studd J, ed. *Progress in Obstetrics and Gynaecology*, Vol. 5. Edinburgh: Churchill Livingstone, 1985; 146–59.

Related topics of interest

Physiology of pregnancy (p. 260)
Puerperal psychosis (p. 298)

RENAL TRACT IN PREGNANCY

Frequency and nocturia are common early on in pregnancy, aggravated by polydipsia, nocturnal fluid shifts when lying in bed and fetal movements impinging upon the bladder. Stress incontinence may occur. The urethra elongates and the bladder becomes more distensible and loses tone leading to larger capacity. There is dilatation and kinking of the ureters (right more than left because of uterine dextrorotation) up to the calyces, which is the result of hormonal dilatation and uterine pressure on the ureters. This notwithstanding there is no marked increase in vesicoureteric reflux in pregnancy, but such factors may exacerbate urinary stasis and infection. The kidneys enlarge by up to 1 cm because of this dilatation, increased GFR and intersitial fluid. The GFR is 60% higher than normal by 16 weeks and remains so until term, and renal plasma flow is 30–50% higher than normal by 20 weeks. Consequently the non-pregnant average values for creatinine and urea of 73 μmol/l and 4.3 mmol/l respectively decrease to average values in the pregnant woman of 51 μmol/l and 3.1 mmol/l. Proteinuria increases, with an upper limit of normal of 300 mg/24 h collection. Plasma albumin declines early in pregnancy and then remains static until term. Any post-partum imaging of the renal tract should be left until at least 12 weeks to allow any changes to resolve.

Asymptomatic bacteriuria

Here true bacteriuria exists without symptoms or signs of an acute urinary tract infection (UTI). True bacteriuria is distinguished from a contaminated specimen on the basis of a fresh midstream urine (MSU) with >100 000 colonies/ml. *E. coli* is the most common organism grown. The frequency is 5% with a prevalence of 1.2%. Up to 40% of such women may have an upper renal tract infection. There is a link between UTI and low birthweight and preterm labour. Reinfection and relapse occur in about 15% of such patients. Antibiotic therapy should be for at least 2 weeks and the urine recultured a week after stopping treatment, and thereafter regularly during pregnancy.

Acute UTI

This may occur as lower or upper tract infection and has been implicated in IUGR, congenital abnormalities, fetal death and premature labour. Lower tract infection affects about 1% of pregnant women. The microbes responsible are those as for asymptomatic bacteriuria. Upper tract infection, i.e. acute pyelonephritis, is the commonest renal complication of pregnancy and has a wide differential diagnosis. Once diagnosed it should be aggressively treated with intravenous antibiotics for 2–3 weeks, initially in a hospital setting. Thereafter patients should have their urine cultured at each antenatal visit. Post-natally an IVU and renal function assessment is warranted.

Pre-existing renal disease in pregnancy

Apart from a tendency for chronic pyelonephritis to recur in at least 20% of cases, most renal tract disease is not adversely affected by pregnancy. Many chronic renal disease patients are hypertensive at conception, although there is a tendency for an exacerbation to occur, particularly in diffuse and focal glomerulonephritis and arteriolar nephrosclerosis. Fifty per cent of renal patients will reveal proteinuria in pregnancy. It may be massive, >3 g/24 h collection, and it may lead to the nephrotic syndrome. Acute renal failure may occur in these women, but it is rare and most will experience only a mild to moderate, reversible decline in function. The GFR is generally lower in these women at the start of pregnancy, but it increases in parallel with the increase seen in non-renal patients. Superimposed pre-eclampsia may well occur, but this diagnosis is hard to make in patients who are proteinuric and hypertensive from the outset. The perinatal mortality rate, preterm delivery rate and small-for-dates baby rate are generally higher in this group. The long-term outlook for renal function after pregnancy in this group is generally good, and any deterioration that does occur is primarily due to the underlying renal lesion rather than the effect of the pregnancy.

Specific entities

Acute glomerulonephritis is a rare complication in pregnancy and is usually initially thought to be pre-eclampsia. SLE patients generally do well if the maternal disease has been in remission for at least 6 months prior to conception, but the outcome can be grave if there is evidence of continued activity and decline in function. Diabetic nephropathy, tubulointerstitial disease and polycystic kidney patients generally also do well, but those with periarteritis nodosa and scleroderma do very poorly and may even die in pregnancy. Renal calculi, mostly calcium based, occur in 0.03–0.35% of pregnancies, and may cause an acute, non-obstetric abdomen in pregnancy. Unilateral nephrectomy for previous calculus disease often leaves the remaining kidney infection prone, and this must be monitored. Pelvic kidneys may be associated with early pregnancy loss due to the associated Müllerian tract anomalies. Women with a single kidney are unaffected by pregnancy. Renal transplant patients have a 40% early pregnancy loss due to spontaneous or therapeutic abortion and ectopic pregnancy. Survival of the pregnancy past 12 weeks is associated with a 90% successful outcome.

Management

Renal patients in pregnancy need to be seen every 2 weeks until 32 weeks and thereafter at weekly intervals. They need baseline and serial renal function testing to detect a decline in function and infection. Any infection must be vigorously pursued and eradicated. The blood pressure must be closely monitored and any pre-eclampsia treated appropriately. The fetus must be observed for growth and well-being in the usual ways. (See Biophysical profiles.) The timing of delivery is generally indicated for obstetric rather than renal reasons, although early induction of labour is advocated by some at 38 weeks as renal disease may be linked to intrauterine fetal death after this gestation. Delivery is best carried out in a tertiary referral centre with full medical, obstetric and neonatal support. A diagnosis of new renal disease in a pregnancy must be fully investigated and followed up by the appropriate specialist team, although the definitive diagnosis may only be made well after delivery. Dialysis patients, despite their anaemia, irregular cycles or amenorrhoea, low libido and potency, are potentially fertile. The diagnosis may not be made until a pregnancy is well established for these very same reasons. Data on the outcome are few, although it is held that most are aborted, either spontaneously or therapeutically. Preterm labour and/or Caesarean section is also held to be the rule in this group. Renal transplant patients ideally have a well-functioning graft and good general health for at least 2 years prior to a pregnancy, no proteinuria or hypertension of note, no graft versus host disease or rejection phenomena, a stable GFR with a plasma creatinine of <180 µmol/l and a daily immunosuppressive regimen of <15 mg of prednisolone and <2 mg/kg azothiaprine. These patients must be treated as very high risk in a pregnancy and be regularly monitored by a physician and an obstetrician. They have a >30% chance of developing pre-eclampsia. Meticulous attention to all parameters of fetal and maternal well-being must be maintained, and in particular decline in function, infection, hypertension, anaemia and growth retardation must be avoided if possible. Vaginal delivery is not contraindicated and Caesarean section should be only for obstetric criteria. Cyclosporin A and azothiaprine are not thought to be teratogenic. Renal transplant patients have a significantly enhanced risk of developing premalignant and malignant genital tract disease.

Further reading

Davison J. Renal disease. In: De Swiet M, ed. *Medical Disorders in Obstetric Practice*, 2nd edn. Oxford: Blackwell Scientific Publications, 1989; 306–407.

Davison JM, Lindheimer MD. Pregnancy and renal disease. In: Studd J, ed. *Progress in Obstetrics and Gynaecology*, Vol. 4. Edinburgh: Churchill Livingstone, 1986; 151–65.

Related topics of interest

REPORT ON CONFIDENTIAL ENQUIRIES INTO MATERNAL DEATHS IN THE UNITED KINGDOM 1991–1993

United Kingdom obstetric audit in the form of The Confidential Enquiries into Maternal Deaths is the longest running series of continuous clinical audit in the world. The reports began in England and Wales in 1952, and the latest report covers the triennium 1991–1993. The report covers, England, Wales, Scotland and Northern Ireland, and analyses 320 maternal deaths. These deaths represent a maternal mortality rate of 9.8 deaths per 100 000 total births, which should be compared with figures of 67.1 in 1955–1957, 33.3 in 1964–1966, 18.2 in 1973–1975 and 9.3 in 1982–1984.

Maternal death

Maternal death is defined as death of a woman during pregnancy or before the 42nd post-partum day. The report also includes late deaths, of which there were 46, which are maternal deaths after 42 post-partum days and less than 1 year from delivery.

Maternal deaths can be divided into three categories:

1. Direct, resulting from obstetric complications of pregnancy, labour and the puerperium, 128 (40%) in the report.

2. Indirect, resulting from pre-existing disease, or from a disease that developed during the pregnancy, and which was aggravated by the pregnancy, 100 (31%) in the report.

3. Fortuitous, resulting from causes not related to or influenced by the pregnancy, 46 (14%) in the report.

The latest report comprises 19 chapters, and includes a chapter devoted to recommendations resulting from the enquiries. The report highlights the need for greater consultant care during pregnancy and labour, and the repeated failure of staff at all levels to appreciate the severity of potential problems.

Causes of maternal death

- Thromboembolism.
- Hypertensive disorders.
- Cardiac disease.

- Ectopic pregnancy.
- Haemorrhage.
- Amniotic fluid embolus.
- Anaesthesia.
- Abortion.

Causes of maternal death in the United Kingdom, 1991–1993			
	Direct	Indirect	Fortuitous
Thrombosis and thromboembolism	35		
Hypertensive disorders of pregnancy	20		
Early pregnancy deaths	18		
Haemorrhage	15		
Amniotic fluid embolism	10		
Genital tract sepsis	9		
Other direct deaths	9		
Anaesthesia	8		
Genital tract trauma	4		
Cardiac disease		37	
Other indirect deaths		63	
Totals	**128**	**100**	
Fortuitous deaths			46
Late deaths	10	23	13
Grand totals	**138**	**123**	**59**
Triennium grand total			**320**

As with CESDI and NCEPOD this report is mandatory reading for all obstetricians and it is hoped that the recommendations are reflected in future reports with improved figures.

Further reading

Report on Confidential Enquiries into Maternal Deaths in the United Kingdom, 1991–1993. HMSO, London, 1996.

Related topics of interest

Confidential Enquiry into Stillbirths and Deaths in Infancy (CESDI) (p. 194)
Ectopic pregnancy (p. 28)
Pre-eclampsia and phaeochromocytoma (p. 270)
Report on the National Confidential Enquiry into Perioperative Deaths (NCEPOD) (p. 122)

RHESUS DISEASE

Red cell isoimmunization, with consequent placental transfer of antibodies, is most commonly due to sensitization of a Rhesus negative mother by red cells positive for the Rhesus antigen, which was discovered by Landsteiner and Wiener in 1940.

Pathology

The Rhesus antigen is produced from a complex area on chromosome 1; at least three genes, C, D and E, are involved. The D antigen appears to be the most clinically relevant, with over 95% of cases of Rhesus incompatibility being due to the D antigen, which is inherited by simple Mendelian principles.

Clinical features

Depending on the degree of haemolysis in the affected fetus, the pregnancy may result in miscarriage, intrauterine death, the birth of a severely hydropic infant with attendant obstetric complications (related to fetal size and fetal distress), neonatal anaemia or jaundice leading to kernicterus.

Prophylaxis against isoimmunization is by injection of anti-D when there is increased risk of feto-maternal haemorrhage e.g. APH or at delivery. Recent recommendations are that anti-D is given to all Rhesus negative pregnant women in the third trimester.

Problems

1. Diagnosis: a history of Rhesus isoimmunization or of features suggestive of isoimmunization may be apparent.

All pregnant women should have serum examined for Rhesus antigen and the presence of antibodies, with repeated examinations for Rhesus negative women.

The fetal Rhesus status may be determined in early pregnancy by chorion villus sampling, but there is a significant risk of abortion.

In affected cases the antibody titre may be measured at regular intervals, originally by direct Coomb's test with dilutional titres; a direct assay is now available.

Repeated amniocentesis may be performed and the bilirubin concentration of amniotic fluid estimated from the change in optical density of the sample at 453 nm wavelength. Results may be plotted on to Liley charts giving an estimation of the severity of the disease based on optical density measurements.

Biophysical examination of the fetus may reveal signs of hydrops on ultrasound, or of fetal distress on CTG or ECG. These methods lead to late diagnosis.

Cordocentesis measures fetal haemoglobin directly and is the most accurate investigation available, but is associated with an abortion rate of 2%.

2. Treatment: this will depend on the degree of haemolysis and the gestation.

Delivery of a mature affected baby is the treatment of choice, premature affected babies may require intrauterine transfusion of O Rh-negative, hepatitis negative and CMV negative donor blood cross-matched with maternal blood, which is also irradiated in some centres.

Transfusion may be intraperitoneal or direct via a fetal vein, such as the umbilical vein.

The timing of transfusion depends on gestation and fetal haematocrit and varies between centres. A haematocrit <25% at, or before, 26 weeks warrants transfusion, also <30% after that gestation.

After birth, treatment depends on the degree of anaemia and jaundice and may include transfusion, exchange transfusion and phototherapy.

Conclusion

With the discovery of the Rhesus factor as the major cause of red cell isoimmunization, the development of passive immunization with anti-D has led to a dramatic decrease in the incidence of Rhesus disease.

Further reading

Fairweather DVI. Rhesus affect. In: Turnbull Sir AC, Chamberlain GC, eds. *Obstetrics.* Edinburgh: Churchill Livingstone, 1989: 503–13.

MacKenzie IZ, Selinger M, Bowell PJ. Management of red cell isoimmunisation in the 1990's. In: Studd J, ed. *Progress in Obstetrics and Gynaecology*, Vol. 9. Edinburgh: Churchill Livingstone, 1991: 31–53.

Related topics of interest

THYROID AND PREGNANCY

The thyroid in pregnancy increases in size as a result of the increase in thyroid blood flow and follicular hyperplasia arising from the increased metabolic demands of pregnancy. There is a rise in total thyroid hormone (T4) level, and triiodothyronine (T3) and thyroid-binding globulin (TBG) also rise as a result of increased hepatic synthesis, in the presence of increased oestrogens. In consequence, the absolute levels of free T4 and free T3 do not change and are the same as for non-pregnant euthyroid women. The free thyroxine index (FTI) remains in the normal non-pregnant range as thyroid hormone uptake declines as TBG increases. There is an increased iodide clearance by the gland, matched by an increased renal iodide clearance. The placenta synthesizes thyroid-like stimulating substances. The thyroid returns to normal 3-6 months after delivery.

Pathology

Pregnancy may mimic both hypothyroidism and hyperthyroidism, e.g. thyroid enlargement, tachycardia, bounding pulses, warm extremities, profound lassitude and excess weight gain. Hyperthyroidism may cause infertility, early spontaneous abortion or recurrent spontaneous abortion. Surgical treatment is rarely called for in pregnancy. Medical treatment with antithyroid drugs is more common. Carbimazole is the drug of choice – 30 mg daily to begin with, thereafter 20 mg/day or less. It may be used in conjunction with a beta blocker to control the symptoms of the disease. Thyroxine may be necessary, with dose titration, to maintain a euthyroid state subsequent to this chemical glandular ablation.

Hypothyroid women are generally infertile. The diagnosis of Hashimoto's autoimmune thyroiditis rests with the finding of thyroid autoantibodies and is treated with increased amounts of thyroxine, whereas subacute thyroiditis will respond to antithyroid drugs and thyroxine.

The fetus

Antithyroid drugs will cross over into the fetal circulation and may cause abortion (up to 2%) or IUGR; they are excreted in breast milk. After delivery the neonate should be closely examined for stigmata of hyperthyroidism or hypothyroidism. Symptomatic neonatal hyperthyroidism may necessitate the use of propranolol. Maternal hyperthyroidism has been associated with increased rates of cerebral palsy.

Endemic goitre is rare in the United Kingdom these days. Congenital hypothyroidism is the result if the pregnancy survives to viability and delivery.

Further reading

Turnbull Sir AC, Chamberlain GC eds. Indexed thyroid references. *Obstetrics.* Edinburgh: Churchill Livingstone, 1989.

Related topic of interest

Immunology of pregnancy (p. 225)

INDEX